rohn

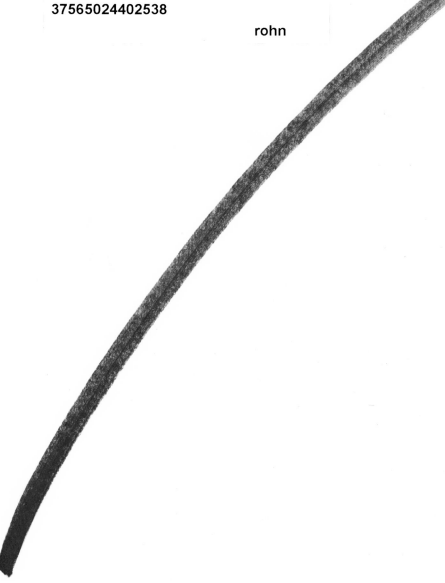

CURING MEDICARE

A volume in the series
THE CULTURE AND POLITICS OF HEALTH CARE WORK

Edited by Suzanne Gordon and Sioban Nelson

Curing Medicare

A Doctor's View on How Our Health Care System Is Failing Older Americans and How We Can Fix It

Andy Lazris, MD
With a foreword by Shannon Brownlee

ILR Press
an imprint of
Cornell University Press
Ithaca and London

Originally published 2014 as *Curing Medicare: One Doctor's View of How
Our Health Care System Is Failing the Elderly and How to Fix It*.

Revised edition first published 2016 by Cornell University Press
Printed in the United States of America

Library of Congress Cataloging-in-Publication Data

Names: Lazris, Andrew, author.
Title: Curing Medicare : a doctor's view on how our health care system is
    failing older Americans and how we can fix it / Andy Lazris ; with a
    foreword by Shannon Brownlee.
Description: Ithaca : ILR Press, an imprint of Cornell University Press,
    2016. I Series: The culture and politics of health care work I Includes
    bibliographical references and index.
Identifiers: LCCN 2015041841 I ISBN 9781501702778 (cloth : alk. paper)
Subjects: LCSH: Medicare. I Older people—Medical care—United States. I
    Geriatrics—United States.
Classification: LCC RA412.3 .L393 2016 I DDC 368.38/200973—dc23
LC record available at http://lccn.loc.gov/2015041841.

Cloth printing   10 9 8 7 6 5 4 3 2 1

To my wonderful wife, Cathy, and my amazing kids, Michael, David, and Rachel. Also to my parents, Yale and Marilyn; my sister, Kim, and brother, Mitch; as well as to Jenny, Marc, Matt, Jacob, Elana, Bryce, Theresa, Jeff, and Mia, and my in-laws Mary and Frank Staropoli. To my running group, who had to hear all my chatter about the book for endless miles: Andres, Paula, and Mike. Finally, to all those I work with, including Pat, Jill, Kathy, Erica, Michelle, Phillip, Libby, Bonnie, and the many administrators, nurses, aides, social workers, therapists, and receptionists who have done so much to make the world I live in better. Thanks to Lou Grimmel for helping me start my practice and for continuing to inspire; to my son Michael for help with research and marketing; and to all the primary-care geriatric doctors out there taking care of their patients with love and expertise in a system that is not always very kind.

CONTENTS

FOREWORD

When Congress passed the Medicare Act in 1965, it was the culmination of one of the most bitter, divisive, and drawn-out battles in congressional history. The need for Medicare legislation was abundantly clear. In 1965, only half of the more than thirteen million Americans over the age of sixty-five had any form of health insurance. Two-thirds had incomes of less than $1,000 a year—a third less than the rest of the population—and many older Americans were living and dying without benefit of any medical care at all. Yet the American Medical Association (AMA), whose principal worry about Medicare was a decline in physician incomes, would spend $50 million over a decade campaigning against what it called at various points a "dangerous device, invented in Germany," a "communist plot," and "socialized medicine." Together with the hospital and insurance industries, the AMA successfully fought off legislation until the 1964 elections brought a majority Democratic Congress and President Lyndon Johnson into office.

Today, Medicare is rightly seen by many as one of the greatest social programs of the twentieth century and a cornerstone of Johnson's "Great Society." It made health care available to millions of elderly citizens, spurred the desegregation of hospitals in the South, and brought down infant mortality rates. Medicare and its sister program Medicaid, which covers the disabled as well as poor children and pregnant women, together provide health insurance coverage to more than eighty million Americans. Yet the politics of Medicare's passage, and the compromises made to appease private insurers, hospitals, and the AMA, set the stage for the rise of the medical industrial complex, to quote the phrase coined by a former editor of the *New England Journal of Medicine,* and can be linked to many of the ills that beset it today.

Among the most tragic of these ills is the way in which elderly, frail, chronically ill Americans are treated by our health care system. When old people who are suffering one or more debilitating chronic illnesses take a fall, feel dizzy, grow confused, or have trouble breathing, they often find themselves on a slippery chute leading straight into the hospital, which has become the default site of care. About a third of U.S. deaths occur in the hospital, despite the fact that the vast majority of Americans say they prefer to die at home.[1] Nearly 17 percent of deaths among Medicare recipients include a stay in the intensive care unit.[2] No matter how fervently patients and their families might wish to avoid invasive treatment as increasing frailty and death approach, and no matter how clearly they have laid out their wishes in an advance directive, the hospital continues to be the site of easiest and first resort.[3] And as Andy Lazris shows in this fine book, nothing a good doctor can say, nothing he can do will change the fact that all too often the way we care for the frail elderly in this country causes untold harm and suffering, and may even be shortening lives.

There are many reasons for this ill-treatment, chief among them a culture of more that assumes there can be no such thing as too much medical intervention. This culture is reinforced by marketing messages from the pharmaceutical industry, which bombard doctors and patients alike. Doctors are rewarded by Medicare (and private insurers) on the basis of so-called "quality" metrics that have been implemented over the last decade in an effort to counter rampant overtreatment but often bear no relationship to the actual health of patients. In this book, much of the author's frustration is aimed at these metrics and the numerous regulatory fixes

Medicare has put in place over the last fifty years to remedy the consequences of compromises that were made to get the legislation passed.

Among the most powerful of these compromises involves the way hospitals are paid. For nearly two decades after Medicare's passage, hospitals were "reimbursed" on a cost-plus basis: each year's payments were based on the costs a hospital reported for several previous years. Like Pentagon suppliers, hospitals were given little incentive to be efficient and every reason to run up the bill. They did this by keeping patients in the hospital for as long as possible, buying new equipment, and expanding the number of beds and staff. Just a year after the legislation was enacted, a report to Congress stated that Medicare's system for paying hospitals "contains no incentives whatsoever for good management and almost begs for poor management."[4]

The legacy of this policy, which lasted until Medicare switched in 1983 to a modified payment model called the diagnostic related group, or DRG, has been the creation of a massive technology-heavy, specialist-centric, hospital-based health care system, with comparatively little investment in community-based primary care. This runs counter to the best models in other high-income countries, where primary care forms the bedrock of health care. In America, hospital services are what the medical industrial complex has been built to offer, and that's what it delivers.[5] Highly invasive "rescue" care is the job for which young doctors and nurses are trained. Not surprisingly, the United States has some of the best, if not *the* best, acute care in the world. If you are going to get in a car accident, do it here. But acute care is often not what the elderly and chronically ill need.

In an effort to address rising rates of hospitalization and unsustainable costs, Medicare has over the years issued a host of regulations and new benefits for beneficiaries, such as hospice and skilled nursing facilities (SNFs), which were intended to encourage the use of lower-cost, non–hospital-based services. It has not quite worked out that way. For example, the use of SNFs and hospice is often associated with *more* hospitalization, not less.[6]

The reasons these regulations and benefits have failed to improve care are many, as Lazris and others have made clear. For example, Medicare part B, which covers such services as physician visits, tests, and physical therapy, does not pay for meaningful home care. The home hospice benefit pays for visits from a health care professional but not for home hospice aids. For beneficiaries who have purchased supplemental insurance, Medicare part A makes a hospital admission the cheapest route even for a complaint that can be remedied at home, a doctor's office, or in the nursing home. Worst of all, for too many elderly people, hospitalization leads to tragic consequences. Statistics, it has been said, are people with the tears wiped away. This book movingly depicts those people: patients who become confused, agitated, and delusional in the hospital; polypharmacy leading to adverse drug reactions; unwanted deaths in the ICU; agitated patients who are "restrained"—doctor code for tied to the bed by the wrists—to prevent them from pulling out tubes or getting out of bed. These are just a few of the ways that aggressive care for the frailest and oldest cause needless suffering and drive up health care costs.

Market fundamentalists may conclude from this book that the problem lies with too much government regulation and that Adam Smith's invisible hand can provide the fix. Let the elderly buy private insurance; for those who are too poor, provide a "defined benefit." But this is no solution. The health care that is paid for through private insurance is no better organized than health care purchased through Medicare. A truly free market would take us back to 1964, when millions suffered and died because they lacked all access to medical treatment.

If Americans are not prepared to simply throw old people to the mercy of the marketplace, and polls suggest that most are not, rising costs will soon force us to grapple with the question of how we want to care for the sickest and most vulnerable among us. For the past fifty years, both Medicare payment policies and the taxpayer dollars that go toward the training of doctors and nurses have supported the expansion of our hospital-centric system while starving the community-based social and medical services that would improve the lives of millions of elderly Americans. We have not built the infrastructure that is needed to deliver the "high touch" care that could allow many more elderly people to age in place in their homes. We waste billions on useless or unwanted hospital care for the elderly, while failing to provide regular meal delivery or aides to help with house cleaning and bathing, simple services that can help an elderly person preserve autonomy and dignity. We are not training health care professionals to talk to patients and families to ensure that the care they receive is in line with their wishes for the declining years of their lives. We have too many specialists in many parts of the country and too few primary care doctors practicing in the community—in part because our teaching hospitals make more money when they train more specialists. The primary care doctors we do have are not rewarded for making house calls and are often too busy to leave their offices in any case.

Shifting toward a community-based health care delivery system will require public investment and massive redirection of money and resources. That's something the $3 trillion behemoth that is U.S. health care will not readily accept, and it will take enormous political will to make it happen. But happen it must. Baby boomers with aging and dying parents are experiencing firsthand the failures of our system. Let's hope self-interest compels them to begin advocating, and soon, for better care for themselves. In the meantime, it is my hope that every policy maker and legislator in the country reads this book. It is not a conservative attack on the system written by a physician who would like to see Medicare disappear. It is a first-hand account from a committed doctor, who sees in the tears that lie behind the statistics the need for a transformed system.

Shannon Brownlee

ACKNOWLEDGMENTS

Thanks to Suzanne Gordon, my editor, who helped me work through the book to make it both stronger and more impactful. Her suggestions and additions were invaluable.

Thanks to Bob Duggan for helping me throughout the entire writing and marketing process, and for being a strong advocate for the book. Thanks to the progressive and forward-thinking organizations to which I belong, including the Lown Institute, the National Physicians Alliance, and the American Medical Directors Association.

Curing Medicare

Introduction

My Boss

Nearly all men die of their remedies and not of their illnesses.
MOLIÈRE, *Le malade imaginaire*, 1673

Recently I gave an educational talk to a group of nurses and aides at a nursing home and assisted-living facility about the dangers of hospitalizing the frail elderly who live in long-term care. I am a certified medical director (CMD), which means that I took courses and underwent additional extensive training to acquire a title that I can tack on after my MD. But most significantly, through my training and subsequent conferences I mastered the regulatory minutiae and Medicare rules that impact much of geriatric medicine in the twenty-first century. I currently direct several assisted-living facilities and retirement communities, as well as a nursing home. When I talk to the nursing staff, I usually focus on a pragmatic area of health care that will alter the way they care for their aged patients.

In this particular talk I distributed a handout enumerating the many pitfalls elderly people may encounter in a hospital, highlighting the lack of efficacy and inherent dangers of hospital care in many circumstances. In fact, as I repeated multiple times in my talk, treating them in the facility itself instead of a hospital is typically more humane and beneficial. The talk went over particularly well, because the nurses and aides understood the futility of hospitalization from their ample experience and enjoyed discussing the topic.

Later that night, however, I got word that one of the nurses who attended the talk had sent a ninety-eight-year-old woman with dementia from the assisted-living facility to the hospital for confusion and weakness. At the hospital the woman became more confused and had to be sedated. Her arm had been poked with needles and she'd been made to undergo a head scan, something that must have been frightening to her. She was also exposed to potentially harmful medicines, dangerous infections, a high likelihood of treatment mistakes, and a hospital that pushes the most aggressive care on elderly people despite a paucity of evidence to support that approach. As is common, they found a urine infection (something fairly ubiquitous in the elderly, to which much illness is ascribed) and they sent her back, not admitting her to the hospital where she may have been tied down and exposed to even more trauma.

I was not surprised that within hours of hearing my talk on hospitalization, a nurse still insisted on sending this confused patient to the hospital for a fairly common medical issue, when I believed that the patient would have been better off staying put and having more gentle care and observation in familiar surroundings. I understood the many forces that conspired to force her to do something that likely she did not think was clinically necessary or even prudent, something we will discuss extensively in this book.

I saw the patient a few days later. She was in a room with other residents with dementia, sitting in a chair, smiling, and clapping her hands. Some of the nursing aides were leading them in a sing-along. At that moment, freed from blood-pressure cuffs, blood sticks, X-ray machines, nursing-home regulatory rules, and handfuls of medicine, my patient was receiving perfect geriatric care. She was socializing, exercising, and using her brain. She was under no stress. She was not exposed to the sting of modern medicine. The dichotomy between her experience at the hospital and what I witnessed now was striking to me. Now she was in the hands of people who knew her and were making her life enjoyable, instead of at the mercy of people who dug into her elderly body trying to find problems and fix them. The former scenario is the very epitome of good geriatric care, while the latter is a geriatrician's nightmare. The former is also cheap and humane, while the latter is horribly expensive, compromising the financial health of our Medicare system and turning patients into unwitting victims of unnecessary and futile aggressive treatment. Unfortunately, it is the latter that is becoming the norm in the treatment of geriatric patients. And the most tragic part is that Medicare itself is financing and encouraging that expensive and ineffective approach.

With this book I hope to demonstrate how our health-care system is failing our oldest and frailest Americans, and how that failure is inextricably tied to Medicare's philosophy and payment structure. My critique is part of a larger social debate that is developing about the goals of modern medicine in particular and the health-care system in general. Many patients, physicians, other health-care professionals, and health-care organizations—including unions, foundations, patient-safety organizations, and politicians—are becoming increasingly concerned about the principles and practices that escalate health-care costs and put patients at risk.

Over the past few years I have read dozens of books warning of the perils of overtreatment for patients of all ages, especially those who are old and frail. Shannon Brownlee's best-selling book *Overtreatment* focuses on the general problem of unnecessary and unsafe medical treatments. Books by Nortin Hadler (*The Last Well Person* and *Rethinking Aging)* and H. Gilbert Welch (*Overdiagnosed)* explore the medical facts regarding many widely accepted tests, medicines, and procedures. Richard Deyo's book *Watch Your Back* zeros in on one particular aspect of the edifice of overtreatment—unnecessary and dangerous treatments for the back pain that cripples millions of Americans—while Gayle Sulik's *Pink Ribbon Blues* demonstrates how the medical establishment can distort health information with detrimental results. In 2015, Stephen Schimpff's *Fixing the Primary Care Crisis* explored how current strategies have thwarted the doctor-patient relationship, and how enabling better doctor-patient discourse at the primary-care level will lead to better care, lower cost, and higher satisfaction with the system. As I finish this book, I have read *Being Mortal*, surgeon Atul Gawande's eloquent plea for a reconsideration of futile treatment at the end of life, and Angelo Volandes's book *The Conversation*, which tries to help patients and physicians navigate discussions that can lead to less aggressive and more appropriate care during terminal illness.

My book is a part of this larger discussion. Its subject is the crisis in primary and geriatric care. I consider this vexing issue by exploring how one of our most critical health-care programs, Medicare, has become one of the most influential proponents of the kind of aggressive, specialist-oriented care that is driving up health-care costs and increasing the suffering of the elderly and their families. After decades of practice and reflection, I have come to this conclusion far more in disappointment than anger (although I certainly have some of both).

In fact, I love the idea of Medicare. I studied it as a history student at Brown University. I believe in its central role in our health-care system. Its creation has saved countless lives and improved the quality of life for all elderly Americans. It provides millions of Americans who would otherwise lack health-care insurance with access to health-care services. As a financing mechanism it is far more efficient than the private insurance that has been one of the primary cost escalators in our system and which encourages fragmentation of, as well as aggressive and inappropriate care for, millions.

But Medicare is far more than a financing mechanism that brings health care to the elderly. As we will see in this book, the Centers for Medicare and Medicaid Services (CMS) promulgates policies and practices that determine the forms of care it will allow and subsequently what kind of care the elderly receive, where they receive it, and who delivers that care. Medicare also serves as a model that many other health insurance companies follow. For instance, once Medicare sets its rates, enforces rules, or implements new programs, most commercial insurances mimic those changes. I have been immersed in the intricacies of Medicare policies and politics for the past twenty-five years. In the course of my career I've read the debates in Congress and among the intellectual elites about its future, listened to politicians and academic giants dissect its flaws, studied Medicare's own solutions to its woes, and read how the lay press perceives its impending collapse and how it may be saved.

Most important, as an internist whose practice has focused on geriatrics, caring for the old, every day I live under the shadow of CMS's rules, regulations, and reimbursement. What I have come to understand is that Medicare has not escaped the imperatives and priorities of the broader American health-care system. Medicare, which Congress created in 1965 to provide health insurance for the elderly, inherited these imperatives and priorities and has—sometimes unwittingly, sometimes deliberately, sometimes out of sheer exhaustion—reinforced these priorities. Some of those who are fighting for a more rational health-care system brandish as their slogan "Medicare for All." As a financing mechanism for a tax-supported national health-care system, this may be a wise idea. As a model of policies and practices that guide the delivery of health-care services to the elderly, it needs to be examined critically. We need to think about the kinds of services and priorities that CMS promotes, whether for the elderly, or potentially for every American, before simply superimposing the Medicare system on a more general model of care.

Because I am a geriatric physician, Medicare controls a huge part of my life. It pays the bills and sets the rules of my practice. I cannot charge more or less than it dictates, I must write notes as it instructs, and even my interactions with families and patients are controlled by its regulations. The problem is that Medicare has been deeply influenced by the kind of contemporary medical thinking that equates aggressive, specialized care with good care, even for patients very advanced in years. That lore has taken root in how Medicare treats its seniors, and prompts our financially strapped national insurance to thrust a large amount of its budget into futile efforts to keep people alive at the end of their lives with the full gamut of technologically advanced medical services. As we will discuss further in this book, physicians in the United States have been taught and "incentivized" to deliver this kind of care. The media has pushed it, and many patients—even some of the oldest—are fueled in their misconception by doctors, the press, drug companies, and the very zeitgeist of the American way of life to believe the false credo that more is better. Others are pushed to be aggressive by Medicare's rules. Hovering over everything is the politics of perception: when Medicare curtails any service, people on both sides of the political aisle cry foul, insinuating that any restriction in Medicare's quest to do everything for everyone is akin to letting our elderly die.

The sad reality is that Medicare has become an active partner in our national obsession with illness. Americans think they are sick and perpetually search for cure and resolution, especially as they age.[1] Their quest for medical answers to the ravages of aging fills them with a heavy dose of stress, merely exacerbating their own decline and dragging the health-care delivery system down with them.[2] The public—from patients and their families to doctors, experts, politicians, and journalists—believe that with enough perseverance, our health-care delivery system is capable of virtually anything, even reversing the ravages of aging. From that perch of false information, and with incentives pushing them, many patients and their families plunge into a sea of aggressive care, often unwittingly.

One could argue that the youngest and most vibrant Medicare recipients, many of whom still work and engage in vigorous activity, may benefit from aggressive care. Plenty of people dispute this claim, and in some cases I agree with them, but I will not address that debate in my book. Most of my subjects are the oldest and sickest of our Medicare patients, and among these, many have dementia, live in assisted-living facilities and nursing homes, and often utilize excessive Medicare resources without deriving any benefit from their "thorough" care. To what would actually help the very old—compassionate care delivered in their own homes—Medicare all too often turns a blind eye, reluctant to assist those who seek dignity and comfort in their quest to stay healthy and active in their later years without being driven into the claws of medical excess.

A century or so ago US medicine evolved from a field dominated by charlatans who dispensed potions and false promises to a distinguished profession led by well-trained practitioners versed in the science of medical care. (See Paul Starr's *The Social Transformation of American Medicine* for an excellent discussion of the history of health care in the United States.) Unfortunately, as medical science advanced, so too did the perception that science and technology could cure everything. More machines, drugs, procedures, and tests sprouted across our medical landscape, and the belief spread that all illness, even the illness of age itself, would fall prey to the ingenuity of medicine. People no longer had to get sick and die. By utilizing all our brilliant resources, by assaulting disease at its roots, we could halt the aging process and begin a trek toward immortality. None of that proved to be true, but the public started to believe it. More specialists emerged, promising more narrowly focused care. More scans, more drugs, and bigger and more sophisticated hospitals proliferated, growing from an errant belief. And into this landscape stepped Medicare, the most expansive leap into health-care delivery ever enacted by the US government.

President Truman was the first to attempt creating a comprehensive, inclusive health-care system, but his effort was ultimately thwarted by the perception, despised in the United States, that his reform would lead to rationing of care.[3] Similar arguments also destroyed President Clinton's attempted reform efforts and emasculated President Obama's Affordable Care Act (ACA). When President Johnson pushed through Medicare in 1965, he too met vigorous opposition from medical and community groups that feared a loss of autonomy for patients and doctors and envisioned Medicare sparking a socialized medical system that would compromise medical standards in the United States, lower the level of excellence in research and care, and lead ultimately to rationing. The AMA (American Medical Association) especially fought to stop Medicare's enactment,[4] something I researched as part of my senior thesis at Brown University. I pored through AMA journals, in which physicians and medical experts predicted doom if Medicare became reality, and I read contemporary articles in newspapers and magazines that mirrored much of the debate we are hearing now regarding health-care reform and its potential to destroy quality through rationing. The AMA actually proposed its own more private insurance plan for the elderly called Eldercare even as it threatened to boycott Medicare and not participate. When it finally did agree to endorse Medicare, the AMA had forced enough concessions from the government, especially with regard to keeping doctors and hospitals strong and independent, that it actually gained financially from the plan's enactment.[5] It is not ironic, then, that the AMA is one of many medical organizations now fighting to keep Medicare intact and largely unchanged, despite its initial opposition to the plan. Doctors and hospitals thrive in Medicare, as Medicare finances the most advanced and aggressive medical care for all elderly Americans. At Medicare's birth such a philosophy seemed both sound and affordable. But the medical profession, and the population it serves, has changed dramatically since 1965.

When Medicare was envisioned, there were far fewer elderly in the United States requiring health care. The population over age sixty-five, before Medicare started caring for them, accounted for about 8 percent of the population, or 12 million people. By 2009 the elderly represented 12.8 percent of the population, nearly tripling to 35 million people. By 2050 the elderly are expected to be 20 percent of the US population, exploding to 88.5 million people. Among the elderly, the very old are proportionately growing faster than any other group. Those over eighty are projected to be the most populous age group by 2050, representing 7.4 percent of the population, or 32.5 million people.[6] Medicare must now serve more and older people than its framers anticipated.

The number of Medicare recipients with diseases of dementia, such as Alzheimer's disease, has also ballooned since the insurance's inception. At the time Medicare was scripted, Alzheimer's was not even identified as a medical condition, and the cost of dementia care was minimal. But as that reality has changed, the cost of such care has accelerated rapidly. Currently 5 million Americans are diagnosed as having Alzheimer's, and that number is expected to reach 7 million by 2025. The cost of caring for those people is estimated at $203 billion, over half of which is paid by Medicare. The total cost of care is expected to reach $1.2 trillion by 2050.[7] In 2015 Medicare spent $112.7 billion caring for people with dementia, constituting almost 20 percent of total expenditure. The cost per recipient incurred by Medicare is $21,585 annually for those with dementia, and $8191 for those without.[8] Currently 61 million Americans care for their ill or disabled family members, many of whom have dementia, spending an average of eighteen hours a week doing so. A quarter of the baby-boom generation provides care for an aging parent.[9] Because Medicare pays so little to help care for people with dementia in their homes, often families have to hospitalize their loved ones out of desperation, something that escalates Medicare costs needlessly. Medicare's framers never considered the consequences of dementia and other debilitating diseases of aging on its model of care.

In addition to the sheer numbers and illnesses of its clients, Medicare's expenses are impacted by changes in health-care delivery since 1965. We are now a medical society dominated by specialists, high-priced tests and procedures, and very expensive hospitals. Compared to 1965, Medicare patients now have at their disposal massive amounts of medical technology that society has embraced as being the most thorough means of assaulting illness and disability. In addition, because from its inception Medicare has focused on and finances hospital care above all else, every American over age sixty-five has access to Medicare A, which pays for hospitalization. The hospital is free for all elderly Americans after a single deductible (approximately $1,000), a cost that is usually paid by their secondary insurance. The hospital remains the center of care for the elderly, the place where older Americans must go when they are too sick to stay at home, when they seek Medicare's payment for round-the-clock nursing and rehabilitation services, and when they want Medicare to pay for certain invasive treatments such as IV fluids and antibiotics. Under Medicare's current payment structure, the frail elderly are pushed into the hospital even when they would prefer to stay at home, despite the peril and price tag that such a journey entails.

Medicare B covers most other services, including doctor's visits, tests, procedures, and certain physical therapy. Americans have to pay a small premium to enroll in Medicare B, and well over 90 percent of Americans have done this. After charging patients a nominal deductible (approximately $150), Medicare B will pay for 80 percent of all services. The vast majority of Americans purchase secondary insurance that will pay the 20 percent of cost that Medicare does not cover. Thus, most elderly Americans, after paying their annual premiums and secondary insurance cost, receive all medical services without charge. Medicare B will not pay for meaningful health care in the home, for home health aides, or for medicines. Often when they get too ill, patients will need to use Medicare A, and that typically requires a stay in the hospital. In its current form, Medicare puts no limits on expensive tests and specialty visits, encourages hospitalization for those most ill, and does not contribute to more palliative care in the home.

The newest incarnation of Medicare, which was enacted in 2006, Medicare D, covers a large part of medication costs for those recipients who pay an annual fee. Already by 2010 the program was costing the federal government $62 billion, or 12 percent of the entire Medicare budget.[10] Congress made two crucial errors in enacting part D. First, it underestimated the cost of the program and how widely it would be used. Second, it explicitly prohibited the government from negotiating with pharmaceutical companies to create a formulary of reasonably priced medicines, a strategy that other federal agencies, such as the Department of Veterans Affairs (VA), have employed to keep costs down. As a result, Medicare D recipients can choose the most expensive brand-name drugs with little restriction and with no competitive price reductions.[11] In a medical landscape cluttered by high-priced drugs that promise the elderly miraculous results, Medicare D has become an albatross that strangles the entire Medicare system.

The result of Medicare's failure to adjust as the world has changed around it has taken a toll on the US economy, placing Medicare under the political microscope as one of the primary drivers of our budget deficit. Although over the past few years the rate of growth of Medicare has slowed, it is still growing and becoming more costly. The financial numbers are staggering. Medicare cost the government $7.1 billion in 1970, $35 billion in 1980, $109.7 billion in 1990, $219 billion in 2000, and $550 billion in 2012.[12] The cost of care escalates for the oldest of Medicare's recipients. In 2011 the per capita cost among Medicare recipients over eighty-five was nearly double the amount spent on younger people ($13,788 versus $7,859). The cost of those who reported they were in poor health was even higher, with the costliest 5 percent of beneficiaries accounting for 40 percent of all Medicare spending. Many of these people are very old, dealing with dementia, and living in institutions.[13] Many are forced into the hospital and encouraged to undergo tests and procedures that are both costly and ineffective. No amount of money can fix their aging bodies, and much of the money spent for their care likely causes more harm, as we will show. A 2013 *Washington Post* article highlighted that in the US medical system, 1 percent of patients exhaust 21 percent of total health-care costs, at a price of $88,000 per person per year.[14] Clearly the sickest Americans, many of whom are not likely to improve despite the money spent on their care, are taxing our system, often for reasons related to Medicare's payment structure.

Can thorough and aggressive medical care help prolong life and improve its quality for our oldest patients? The very idea that overutilization of health care leads to improved outcomes has been debunked repeatedly, something we will explore extensively in this book.[15] We in the geriatric field know it innately; our very souls are watered by the knowledge that more is less, and that aggressive care can be deleterious care. When one studies the literature it becomes apparent that there is a paucity of data specifically relevant to our oldest patients, many of whom have multiple illnesses and are on a plethora of medicines.[16] So, often erroneously, we extrapolate data from younger patients, or we accept assumptions that have been hammered into our heads, that all diseases should be eradicated, and that our society is blessed with an abundance of life-saving treatments. In fact, as little as 15 percent of what doctors do is backed up by valid evidence that supports its efficacy.[17] And thus we send our oldest and frailest patients on a journey that is costly both to them and to society with little evidence to back us up.

Many books and studies have explored the false notion that aggressive care leads to improved outcome in the elderly, and I have been lucky enough to be able to use them as resources.[18]

But the crux of my argument flows from my own experience and that of my colleagues. While medical literature can help guide us to make sensible decisions, most of us who practice medicine every day have become skeptical as to the validity of what we read in journals. We know that many studies are financed by pharmaceutical companies and special interest groups, that the overly screened subjects accepted into such studies look nothing like the more complicated patients we see every day, and that the conclusions are subject to many interpretations. We also have seen studies touting the benefits of a drug or treatment, only to be completely reversed some years later. When I was a medical student it was considered standard care to treat women with estrogen after menopause, and it was deemed dangerous to treat patients with failing hearts (congestive heart failure) with a class of drugs called beta-blockers. Studies and literature supported such suppositions, academic physicians assured us of their validity, and clinical pathways enshrined such beliefs as gospel. Well, some years later, new studies emerged, and now it is bad practice to give women estrogen after menopause and to deny patients with congestive heart failure beta-blocker drugs.

There are so many examples where science and dogma are turned on their heads, leaving us doctors to ascertain reality for ourselves. I have seen academics and physicians interpret a single study to argue opposite points, showing me that the literature is far less scientific and objective than we are led to believe. Finally, few large studies focus on the frail elderly among their subjects, and those are the people most vulnerable to the sting of aggressive care. Hence, while I frequently cite the literature that is out there, in this book I rely on my own experience as a geriatric doctor to reach many of my conclusions.

My own career as a doctor has demonstrated to me the futility of pursuing excessively thorough care for many elderly patients, while revealing to me the wall Medicare has enacted that prevents us from offering our patients a more sensible and economical alternative. My career started in a small town called Taunton, and that two-year experience opened my eyes wide to what is wrong with our current Medicare system. Taunton was a world unto itself. Small and isolated in the bog-filled serenity of southeastern Massachusetts, with a population made up of many ethnic Portuguese who had been there for generations, Taunton was home to large numbers of working-class families who rarely moved away. And although they lived half an hour away from the medical meccas of Boston and Providence, most of my patients refused to travel that far; they preferred little

Morton Hospital with six beds in a room and their local doctors. They trusted us, they listened to us, they respected us, and they treated us with unfettered kindness.

In Taunton in those days my patients understood the limits of medical intervention. They did not chase medical miracles or rely on the promises made by aggressive doctors, pharmaceuticals, and the press. Compared to the well-educated enclaves in which I practiced subsequently, my Taunton patients understood the aging process and based their decisions on common sense and dignity. These were the smartest group of patients with whom I have ever worked.

Often on my way home to East Providence I made home visits, where I was greeted with a hug and a smile, never a list of demands or piles of Internet articles. One day I stopped to see an elderly Portuguese woman with moderate dementia. She lived in a two-story colonial house that was older than she was, cuddled upstairs in a small bedroom with a hospital bed and a large, metal lifting mechanism (called a Hoyer Lift) next to some old upholstered furniture and a nightstand. Grandkids ran in and out, up and down; any number of them visited the house regularly. Some children lived in the house, many others lived nearby, all congregated here on the days I arrived.

Whenever I saw Mrs. A. she smiled and held my hands gently. She spoke a few words in Portuguese that her daughters translated for me, typically general pleasantries rather than anything of particular substance. I would listen as she or her daughters expressed any concerns. We reviewed her medicines, stopping any that seemed no longer needed or not beneficial. I took her blood pressure, and listened to her heart and lungs, a step required of all of us in the medical field. After my brief visit Mrs. A. thanked me profoundly, typically with a kiss on the cheek, after which her daughter pushed something on me, such as homemade sweet bread or a box of candy. I always left elated, although part of my brain questioned the significance of the service I provided or the wisdom of Medicare paying me for doing so little.

One dreary winter day I stopped by her house at the behest of one of her daughters. After our traditional greetings, I noticed that Mrs. A.'s eyes were yellow. She was scratching herself, something that proved to be her daughter's main concern that day. She still smiled, and the stomping and laughter of children had not faded one bit. I examined her. She had a large liver protruding down to her groin, and she was severely jaundiced. I was concerned.

I took her daughter aside. "Your mom has something serious going on," I told her. "She has jaundice. We may need to do some tests."

The daughter smiled. "My mother is eighty-five years old," she said. "If we could just give her something for her itching. She seems so uncomfortable."

"But it could be treatable," I went on. "Maybe it's a gallstone. Or a resectable cancer."

The daughter put her hands on my shoulder. "She is eighty-five," she repeated, with a smile that shined with absolute serenity and conviction. "I don't want to put her through all those tests. But I would like her not to be so uncomfortable, if that is even possible. You tell us what is best."

I nodded and gave her both an antihistamine for the itching and some Questran powder that worked particularly well for the jaundice itch (although very constipating, as I warned the daughter). The daughter stepped to another room for a moment, and returned with a bottle of wine in a woven basket casing. "Take this," she said. "And thank you. My mother feels so much better after your visits. And so does the whole family. Thank you so much." It was as if the daughter knew that this would be my final visit.

Mrs. A. died many months later, comfortable and surrounded by her family.

If only all of our country followed the sensible script of Mrs. A. and many of my other patients in Taunton in those days. She charged Medicare no more than the cost of a few of my visits and some rented medical supplies. Probably less than a thousand dollars. And all this for the perfect ending to a relatively stress-free aging process.

Contrast that to an adult child who chided me for not checking her eighty-plus-year-old dad's PSA blood test, and when she did bring him to a urologist at a major academic medical center to perform that test, and it showed that he had prostate cancer, she graced me with several instructional notes about how his new squadron of doctors were actually doing something for her dad, rather than neglecting him as I did. After a multitude of tests, biopsies, scans, treatments, and visits to the most brilliant minds at a renowned hospital far from his home, my once carefree patient became consumed by stress, and finally did die, of a heart attack, not anything to do with his PSA. After which his child said: "At least I know that they were thorough in their treatment of my dad and we did all we could to get him well." She would have had it no other way. Tens of thousands of dollars later, dollars paid by Medicare, her father died of stress, likely precipitated by the very misguided pursuit that Medicare financed.

In any given week I may encounter a patient or family member who demands unreasonable tests, treatments, hospitalizations, specialist visits, and impossible answers for the ravages of aging in patients little different from Mrs. A. Instead of loving kindness and an acceptance of aging, they conjure incessant stress for themselves, their loved ones, and me and my staff by trying to achieve the impossible. On any given day I will encounter many more patients and families who prefer to live the life of Mrs. A., be kept comfortable, be on fewer medicines, and have fewer tests, but who are pushed reluctantly in the direction of aggressive care by a medical system, a society, and an insurance that enables and encourages excess.

Whenever I hear about proposals to ameliorate our society's excessive consumption of medical care, I find that many reformers ascribe blame to doctors who both profit from and relish a health-care system that is fueled by excess. Such reformers concoct ingenious theories that contend that by tying physician salary to performance and not to fee-for-service somehow patients will no longer be allowed to abuse services. But in my career I have seen it from a different angle. Many primary-care doctors do their best to stop older patients from pursuing aggressive care, only to be met by a system that not only pays for that care but encourages it. In fact, we as primary-care physicians are not given the power or authority to slow the overuse of resources. Medicare encourages patients and families to be aggressive, and it pays specialists and hospitals generously to be aggressive; primary-care providers are often sidelined while needlessly aggressive care is administered.

It is thus not surprising that some of my most frail patients, and their families, often demand "thorough" care for many reasons. One is financial; as we will discuss, under Medicare's rules it is often much less expensive for them to get aggressive medical treatment than to be conservative and compassionate, even if it costs Medicare substantially more and the outcomes of such care may be worse. But just as important, many of my oldest patients, and their families who ultimately make the decisions about their welfare, believe in aggressive care. They have been inundated by the idea that more is better at any age, that numbers need to be fixed, that a cure is out there if only they pursue it. Even those who are skeptical are forced to live in a society where everyone else is telling them to be aggressive. When conservatives talk about death panels, and liberals declare that any restrictions on Medicare spending is akin to killing people, it is difficult for anyone to make rational decisions.

One of my good friends, a fellow geriatric physician, lamented to me the other day about a situation involving a patient of his, Mrs. L., who was far more ill than Mrs. A had been. She was old and had dementia, although independent until only recently when a series of medical insults had left her weak and confined to a nursing home. She now relied on kidney dialysis and artificial food to keep her alive. My friend was appalled to learn that her family sought to pursue every option and treatment to maintain her life at all costs, even though several doctors had advised them otherwise. "She was living on her own just a few months ago," her family members said. My friend spent hours of unreimbursed time talking to doctors, reviewing notes, and reasoning with her children. But they persevered. "She was living on her own just a few months ago." They could not get past that fact. And the more my friend pushed to keep her comfortable, the more they resisted him. So they found a new doctor, one willing to perform dialysis on a woman who could no longer feed herself or talk, dialysis that is well reimbursed by Medicare. And they found a new nursing home willing to endorse their aggressive approach to care.

These were educated adult children. One was a nurse. But how little they understood the aging process, and how little they realized what older people really desire in their last months! Over 70 percent of elderly say they want to die at home, not in a hospital.[19] But there is a very sharp divide between the more palliative approach that most elderly seek and how aggressively their families, doctors, and the system treat them.[20] Many families are peering through a jaded lens. They love their mom so much that they just want to keep her alive and wish for a miracle, the miracle of reversing age and returning her to her healthy state when she lived alone. The illusion of turning back the clock with aggressive care is alluring but often deceptive. In the elderly, it only takes one illness to trigger a chain reaction in the body that decimates it. Healthy three months ago and dialysis dependent now does not mean a mere blip has occurred. It is, rather, one of the consequences of aging, the end-stage of a process that was accelerating beneath the surface and then exploded to its tragic conclusion. But fantasy overtakes their thoughts. Medicare pays the bills. And their mom pays the price.

Many of my patients squander tens of thousands of Medicare dollars in their last months of life, clinging to a quixotic hope that cure is possible if they push hard enough and spend enough money. End-of-life expenses, in fact, are one of the primary drivers of medical costs for the elderly. Twenty-five percent of total Medicare expenses finance end-of-life care, care that accomplishes nothing but painfully prolonging the inevitable. Incredibly, with the endorsement of Medicare, the health-care profession unleashes the full force of its medical resources at problems that are not fixable and merely lead to death.[21] While only a negligible amount of Medicare funds are spent on helping people like Mrs. A. stay comfortable in their home where they can receive appropriate medical care, Medicare spends a quarter of its entire budget trying to save people who are not savable and who usually do not want to be "saved."

Although a majority of elderly people want to die at home with comfort, only a fifth of them actually achieve that goal. Fifty percent die in a hospital, and 40 percent of those are in intensive care units where they will likely be sedated or have their arms tied down. Few elderly elect to be treated with such flagrantly ineffective aggression in their final days and months, but many forces, including the harsh reality of Medicare, push them where they do not want to be. Another 30 percent of the elderly die in nursing homes, often explicitly against their wishes, forced to bow to the financial realities of our current geriatric health-care system.[22]

In the following pages we will explore Medicare's continued advocacy of aggressive medical care despite suffocating costs and poor outcomes from that approach, and will examine why Medicare seems unable to control that excess or redefine geriatric medical care so that it can sensibly address the changing population that it serves. This book is not an assault on Medicare, which is an invaluable program that has transformed the care of our elderly, but rather is a critical analysis of how Medicare's priorities may be leading to the very poor and expensive care that its reformers seek to change. As a primary-care doctor I am immersed in Medicare daily. I see how it impacts my ability to care for patients and my patients' ability to access the care they want for themselves. In fact, the very reason I wrote this book is because I value Medicare, and I seek to lend a voice to those who are calling for common-sense changes. As we will see, Medicare in its current incarnation is both unsustainable and counterproductive in the quest to achieve the high-quality cost-effective health care that most doctors and their patients crave. Its reforms, many of which have driven doctors out of the system and which stymie my ability to care for my patients every day, are also leading us down a road no less rosy than the system they are trying to repair. In fact, to paraphrase an almost Orwellian zinger that distresses every primary-care doctor I know, we are now being implored to practice "quality" and "value" care using mechanisms that are the very antithesis of quality and value; the individuality of each patient is lost in the homogenization of health-care delivery that relies on quantifiable metrics that doctors must spend much of their time documenting in computers rather than looking patients in the eyes and having more meaningful conversations. If we are going to really cure Medicare, we must move our gaze to the doctor's office and see how the current system and its complex array of reforms color the interaction between doctor and patient, between patient and the health-care-delivery system, between quality geriatric care and the realities of what Medicare offers its recipients. When we look at it in that context, I believe we are moving in a very dangerous direction, but one that can be easily righted with the input of doctors and patients rather than pundits and professional reformers.

Unless we curb the dangerous folly of aggressive care in our oldest residents, unless we realize that with age comes a decline that no amount of dollars will curtail, unless we stop financing a medical quest that leads to nothing more than the very death it is attempting to stop, and unless we provide our elderly with the comfort and dignity that the vast majority of them seek, then Medicare will not persevere. Few of the innovations concocted by CMS or the Medicare reformers confront that reality. Few of them are proposing feasible means of helping Mrs. A.'s experience become the norm. But that should be our ultimate goal.

1

DEFINING QUALITY

The Quest for Numerical Perfection

> Everyone dies of something. Every time a new complication develops, the doctor will assign it a name, giving you another diagnosis. . . . Each diagnosis has a potential treatment, which the doctors will dutifully tell you about— if you haven't already looked it up on line.
>
> IRA BYOCK, *The Best Care Possible*

The pharmaceutical industry has thrived in this country because people believe that medicines are both essential and useful to repair a variety of dangerous and bothersome conditions, something that is especially true in the elderly. Whether treating aberrant numbers (blood pressure, cholesterol, sugar, etc.) or helping to resolve nuisance conditions like urinary incontinence and confusion, drugs flood our elderly patients' bodies. But many medications have dubious efficacy and can be frankly dangerous. Often they are used to treat problems that do not meaningfully improve, and more often they instigate troublesome symptoms, drug interactions, and harmful side effects.

Medicare does not itself compel patients to take more medicines; our national drug obsession is a much more complex phenomenon than can be ascribed simply to Medicare. But especially since the advent of Medicare D and the adaption of clinical performance measures (labeled as quality indicators by CMS) to grade doctor quality, Medicare is playing a larger role in encouraging and financing excessive medication use. And as we discussed, Medicare D places minimal restrictions on what drugs patients can take, and does not negotiate with pharmaceutical companies to secure medicines that are lower in cost but equally efficacious. Said one doctor who has studied this problem: "If the government's real goal were to increase senior citizens' access to the most effective medicine, its first step would have been to determine the best care based on the best scientific evidence available, helping patients and doctors to make informed decisions. Instead, the medicine prescription drug bill simply opens the public coffers to pay the price for expensive brand name drugs."[1]

As significantly, Medicare as part of its reform effort is grading doctors based on the quality of their care, something that also can actually lead to more medication use. Through two programs primarily—the Physician Quality Reporting System (PQRS) and Accountable Care Organizations (ACOs), both of which we will discuss in detail later—Medicare is compelling doctors to produce evidence that they are following quality indicators as defined by CMS. We as physicians are required to complete an established set of questions, many of which have little relevance to our particular patients, and to demonstrate that we are in compliance with a variety of such indicators, something that will eventually help determine some of what we are paid. It is felt that such pay-for-performance strategies will help doctors practice better medicine and save the system money. It is a laborious and expensive process for us, and often it pushes us to mindlessly fill out scripted checklists when our time could be better spent having meaningful discussions with our patients. Since every elderly patient has a unique set of wants and needs, and each one offers unique challenges that make templated responses virtually useless, Medicare's attempt to impose quality standards on us yields more busywork than meaningful change.

Quality indicators have another dark side, one that can increase unnecessary testing and treatment in the elderly. By forcing us to comply with specific standards, Medicare expects us to order tests and prescribe drugs that we, and our patients, may not believe to be beneficial. By tying the quality of our care (and ultimately a portion of our salary) to the achievement of those standards, Medicare is pushing us to act in a way that may actually be counterproductive to quality care. Many indicators are designed to persuade doctors to evaluate and treat abnormal numbers. High blood pressure, high cholesterol, high sugars, abnormal bone density results, low heart ejection fraction, irregular heart rhythms—all of these have specific guidelines that script what is deemed to be appropriate testing and treatment. To be fair, many of Medicare's quality indicators are more reasonable than other clinical-practice guidelines, many of which seek aggressive care for virtually every abnormal number in the elderly. But virtually none of Medicare's quality guidelines encourage doctors to *avoid* testing for and treating these abnormal numbers even in the very oldest of our patients; at best, they encourage some testing and treating, and are silent about overtreatment. Just how important is it to treat abnormal numbers in the elderly? That is the crux of what we have to explore, for its answer illuminates much of what is wrong with Medicare and how to fix it.

Numbers

As an internal-medicine resident at the University of Virginia, I spent time in a rural clinic in Orange County working with two excellent doctors. One day they sent me to see a farmer who was in his mid-90s and still worked his farm independently. When I saw the man he seemed strong and young, very calm, fairly sharp, and nimble on his feet. I examined him and found nothing particularly wrong except for his blood pressure, which was close to 220/110 from my recollection. To me this finding was startling. I rechecked it a few times, and the results did not change. The man took no medicines and had no serious medical problems. He felt very well.

I talked to one of the clinic doctors and insisted that we treat the man for his dangerously elevated blood pressure. We had all read the new SHEP (Systolic Hypertension in the Elderly) study that demonstrated the dangers of high blood pressure in the elderly,[2] and thus we needed to be more vigilant in treating pressure elevations among our older patients. The doctor bucked, but I convinced him to allow me to use a very mild blood pressure medicine, and the patient agreed. I told him I would go out there next week and check the pressure again. Well, next week never came. Several days after starting the medicine, the man died. Coincidence? Unlikely. My guess, now that I have more extensive real-life experience with the elderly, is that the man had very narrow arteries to his heart and brain and kidneys, and he needed every bit of that high blood pressure to keep the blood flowing to his vital organs. In fact, his body's natural auto regulation system probably pushed that pressure up to keep him alive. When I gave him a pill to make his numbers look better, I unintentionally dismantled his body's coping mechanism by decreasing that necessary pressure and thus instigated his demise.

This is not an isolated event. Number obsession has reached a fever pitch among the elderly and those who care for them. Numbers are everything, even if we are not quite sure what those numbers should be for each individual. As one doctor states in his book on medical excess: America's elderly know their numbers "and are hell bent to be normal."[3] It may be blood pressure, pulse, sugar, cholesterol, kidney function, bone density, thyroid level, blood count, vitamin levels; there are dozens of numbers that can be measured, fussed over, and fixed with medicines. As people age, their numbers deteriorate and diverge from what is deemed "normal"; the more we look, the more we will find, and the more medicine we will need to dispense to fix.

We know from science and experience that the aggressive treatment of numerical abnormalities in the elderly, especially in conditions like diabetes and hypertension, frequently causes side effects, worsening physical and mental function, and an impaired quality of life without extending lifespan or even preventing major adverse outcomes (such as strokes, heart attacks, and cancer) in a measurably significant way. Medicines can fix numbers, but rarely do they improve a geriatric patient's life. In fact, the more we toss into an elderly body, the more interactions and complications will occur. As we will see, low numbers are typically much more immediately dangerous than high ones; I have seen many more people injured and even killed by aggressive treatment that drops their numbers than by benign neglect. But such a reality does not deter the US medical community from employing an array of medications in pursuit of numerical perfection. If the lore of what defines quality medical care starts anywhere, it is in the theater of medications, where numbers are perceived to be beacons, pills are touted as saviors, and those who push the pills and fix the numbers are our medical saints.

I am frequently told by my patients, and those caring for them, that I have to be more vigilant in monitoring and fixing numbers. Physical therapists and home care nurses e-mail me about blood pressures or sugars that are too high; they often have an alarmist tone when they convey the information, expecting me to intervene quickly. Nursing homes, as we will see, measure and expect immediate treatment for an infinitude of numbers, from thyroid levels to blood pressures, sugars, and a large variety of labs. My patients see specialists, emergency room doctors, and even family members who frighten them about their abnormal numbers. Often these abnormal numbers are merely blips, the results of tests taken at inopportune times when patients are in pain, stressed, ill. Sometimes the numbers are not even very high, but they have crossed some imaginary line between normal and dangerous. The assumption by many who contact me is that once that line is crossed, then a stroke or heart attack or perhaps even death is imminent.

Since numbers can be easily measured, and since so many of them can be "fixed" with medicines, patients often swallow handfuls of pills to push their numbers back to the acceptable side of normal, after which they can be monitored in a variety of ways to ensure the numbers stay in line. And if the numbers start to migrate away from what we have deemed to be normal, more medicines and tests will naturally flow through their frail bodies. But what are normal numbers for the elderly, and does fixing abnormal numbers impart any meaningful clinical benefit to our patients?

We can measure numbers many ways. Tests, labs, vital signs: for every patient, we can compile numbers that come to define them. Then we label our patients with diseases that correspond to their errant numbers. They may have high blood pressure, high cholesterol, diabetes, osteoporosis, hypothyroidism, anemia, dementia, and one of any number of conditions that we can treat and then monitor through copious lifelong testing. In my practice the pursuit of numerical excellence is one of the primary reasons patients see me and an army of specialists on a regular basis. Many doctors who have studied our health-care system believe that the medical community is intentionally manufacturing disease by using these numbers because the medical community thrives when more people are sick. Some state that we are turning aging itself into a disease.[4] Locating a number that equates to an illness and that can be altered with medicine is seems to many people like a productive use of medical science these days.

To best assess the value of measuring and improving numbers in our elderly patients we have only two tools: experience and scientific investigations. The former is a subjective means of assessment that doctors like me utilize based on what years of practicing medicine have taught us, while the latter is alleged to be more objective and universally applicable. The truth is that most studies done on medications do not involve older people, as elderly patients typically are excluded from medication studies.[5] The studies that do have an older cohort rarely involve elderly participants on multiple medicines and with numerous medical problems resembling the majority of older patients for whom I care. Also, most studies are sponsored by drug companies, and when the results of those studies diverge from what the pharmaceuticals desire, the studies are not published.[6] Thus, when we assess the impact of disease and medication on older patients, we are using very little data that is reliable and meaningful.

When we do evaluate studies about numbers and the medicines used to treat those numbers, we must be aware of a very important nuance in the statistical presentation of data, something of which I have only recently become aware in my medical career. Most studies report their results in terms of *relative risk and benefit*. Those numbers could seem very impressive and make a test or treatment appear much more significant than it really is clinically. *Absolute risk and benefit*, however, is a much more revealing number, although rarely reported in the press or medical literature. In addition, it is important that the endpoint of a study reveals a *clinically significant* result. For instance, we do not care if a certain drug improves someone's number; we do care if the drug, by improving the number, helps them be healthier or live longer. Pharmaceutical companies that sell medicines and sponsor studies, medical researchers who gain prominence from demonstrating significant findings from their studies, and even members of the medical community who seek justification for aggressively labeling and treating disease all rely on the allure of relative risk. A small risk to a patient who has an abnormal number (such as high blood pressure), or a small improvement in the patient's health from fixing that number, can be magnified into what seems to be a huge benefit when results are conveyed by relative risk and benefit rather than absolute risk and benefit.

Consider that a lottery in this country has a huge payoff, and you learn that there is a fivefold higher chance of winning if you buy a ticket in Ohio instead of Maryland, where you live. Is it worth flying to Ohio to buy some tickets? The relative chance of winning in Ohio is five times higher, or 500 percent better, than if you purchase a ticket in Maryland, an impressive number and perhaps worthy of a plane ticket. That is relative benefit. But the absolute benefit is much less impressive. If the chance of winning in Maryland is one in ten million, and the chance of winning in Ohio is five in ten million, then the absolute benefit of traveling to Ohio is a four in ten million increased chance of winning, a much less appealing advantage. A five-times relative benefit is really a four-in-ten-million absolute benefit. Thus, although in medical literature we hear almost exclusively about the relative benefit and risk of certain medicines and treatments, that number typically obscures the more relevant truth revealed by absolute risk and benefit.

It is important, then, to evaluate certain clinical situations where medicines are used to fix abnormal numbers in the elderly and to ascertain whether, in absolute terms, such interventions are justified. We also need to determine whether the risks of treating those numbers in the elderly are, in absolute terms, of concern to us. Medicare and the ACA, among other groups, are trying to assess and grade physician quality by tying it to the measurement and fixing of numbers and various medical conditions. This is being touted as a major thrust of reform: paying doctors for quality performance is perceived to be a revolutionary means of saving Medicare. But the validity of such an approach lies hidden in the numbers themselves. The question is: Can we achieve improved health-care outcomes in the elderly at a reduced cost by measuring and fixing numbers through models such as Medicare's quality indicators? The answer to that question reveals a deeply rooted flaw in our geriatric health-care delivery system, a flaw that has blinded many of those who are now trying to reform Medicare, and one that we will explore throughout this book.

The Case of A-fib

Medicare Quality Indicators state that all people over age 18 who are deemed to be high risk for stroke by specified criteria [which include virtually all of the elderly] *should take Warfarin or a similar anticoagulant.*[7]

The treatment of atrial fibrillation (A-fib) with warfarin (brand name Coumadin) is a good illustration of how relative risk can be a misleading means of evaluating a treatment. A-fib is a condition common in the elderly where the heart beats irregularly and rapidly. The primary difficulty with A-fib is that clots can accumulate in the heart and cause strokes. To prevent this complication, doctors place patients on blood thinners such as warfarin, an old rat poison that prevents clots from developing. In fact, people with A-fib on warfarin have 50 percent fewer strokes than do people with A-fib on aspirin.[8] Because of such impressive results, virtually all doctors recommend the use of warfarin in their older patients. Its use is standard care and it is part of every clinical performance measure to which doctors are supposed to adhere. For most of my career, I never questioned its unassailable necessity; after all, why risk a stroke when there is such an effective treatment available?

But numbers can be deceptive. Fifty percent reduction is a relative benefit. In fact, the chance of an older person with A-fib getting a stroke is close to 6 percent a year. With aspirin that number moves down toward 4 percent. With warfarin that number is closer to 2 percent.[9] True, warfarin confers a 50 percent risk reduction compared to aspirin, but that is because it cuts the risk of stroke in half compared to aspirin, reducing it from 2.5 percent with aspirin to 1.4 percent with warfarin.[10] Also, as many as half the strokes that occur are minor and leave no lasting effects, so the clinically relevant improvement is half of those numbers, or a 6/1000 decrease in the number of disabling strokes in people who take warfarin instead of aspirin. That is the absolute risk reduction. Looking at it another way, there is a 99.3 percent chance of averting a clinically relevant stroke with warfarin, and a 98.7 percent chance of averting a stroke with aspirin. When my patients hear about a 50 percent reduction in stroke, they are petrified about using aspirin instead of warfarin, despite their fears of warfarin. When I tell my patients about the absolute risk reduction, however, many of them prefer to take their chances and use aspirin, especially my patients who are older and are on many other medicines.

Why not just use warfarin? Major strokes can be devastating, so even a small risk reduction can be significant. The problem is that warfarin is not a benign drug. It interacts with virtually every medicine and food, from tea, to Tylenol, to a dinner salad. Patients must check their blood levels frequently; failure to do so could result in either ineffective doses or toxic doses. Patients on warfarin bleed more, sometimes dangerously so, especially if they fall down, and especially if they are over eighty. Studies suggest that the risk of serious bleeding ranges from 4 to 7 percent (40–70/1000) of patients each year,[11] which far exceeds the benefit of taking warfarin in many cases. The risk of bleeding in the brain alone, which is another form of stroke (hemorrhagic stroke) is 0.6 percent (6/1000) higher in people taking warfarin than those who take aspirin for A-fib,[12] meaning that almost the entire benefit of warfarin in reducing stroke is erased by the increased risk of a brain bleed, both of which can similarly disable a patient.

For some patients, being on warfarin is like having a leash around their necks; every illness they have, everything they put in their mouths, every medication change or new vitamin they take, every change in their behavior, every time they trip or bump their heads, every bruise or nosebleed, forces them to be aware of their warfarin, check their blood levels, talk to their doctors, make adjustments in dose, or even go to the hospital. To many of my patients, the stress of being on warfarin is probably more likely to cause them a stroke than any risk reduction the drug may incur. And warfarin itself can cause other problems directly, even an increase in the rate of osteoporotic fractures.[13] There are newer, more expensive drugs that have replaced warfarin with similar risk reduction and without the need to check labs incessantly. But these too have side effects that are substantial, not the least of which is the inability to reverse the drug's effect for several days should a bleed occur. The use of anticoagulants such as warfarin in A-fib demonstrates how people use relative risk to exaggerate the importance of employing certain aggressive interventions in older people even when the true efficacy is very small and the potential harm not insignificant. Still, every clinical guideline, including Medicare's quality indicators, assumes that warfarin (or its equivalent) is an absolute necessity for eligible A-fib patients. Failure to use it is construed as a measure of poor quality care. If I discuss the pros and cons of warfarin treatment with a patient, and she chooses to use aspirin instead, I will have failed Medicare's quality indicator. Blindly following protocol, regardless of my individual patient's wants or needs, and regardless of what is best for that particular patient, is regarded as quality care.

The overuse of warfarin is illustrative of our obsession with numbers and how that obsession in the elderly can be deleterious. Measuring warfarin levels by blood provides a number called the international normalized ration, or INR. People on warfarin are advised to maintain their INR within a narrow therapeutic window; if the number is too low they can have a stroke, and if it is too high they can bleed. Given that in many of my patients even a gust of wind seems to impact their INR, the fluctuations of INR are so wide that one cannot reliably know the value from day to day. However, my patients, or their families, are so focused on that number, so convinced that even a slight deviation from the norm will portend disaster, that they alter their lives dramatically to assure that the number remains good, often checking themselves more often than is required and refusing to eat foods they enjoy. Worse than that, many doctors who monitor their warfarin are just as fixated on the number, and will do whatever is necessary to make sure that number stays within its narrow acceptable range, further adding to the stress that warfarin inflicts on its users.

I have dementia patients in nursing homes on warfarin, elderly patients who fall, patients who cannot move or see, others who are on so many other medicines that their levels bounce everywhere. They will not stop this drug, so convinced are they that it is absolutely necessary to save them from a horrible stroke, a conviction reinforced by their doctors, their families, the lay press, and the deceiving relative risk improvement that the drug offers. The drug itself becomes a disease. No one seems to really care just how minimally Coumadin actually helps people stay healthy and how dangerous it can potentially be. They just care about the number. That has become the new marker of quality care.

Hypertension

Medicare Quality Indicators indicate that blood pressure should be kept below 140/90 in patients under the age of ninety. [That number is 120/70 in my ACO's quality indicators]. *Any such patients diagnosed as having hypertension should be on an aspirin, be on a statin cholesterol medicine if LDL cholesterol is elevated, have annual blood and urine kidney testing, have regular testing for diabetes, and should have their blood pressure treated.*[14]

Blood pressure is another number that causes high levels of concern and fear among my elderly patients. Many are convinced that any bump in their pressure means that a stroke is imminent. Many of my patients check their pressure multiple times a day and make graphs and charts, trying to find patterns so they can ascertain methods of keeping the numbers normal. Those who live in nursing homes or with their family, who are having physical therapy or see another doctor, have their numbers checked often as well, frequently contacting me in distress that, even for a single reading, the number is dangerously high. And all of this is based on a number derived from a very imprecise blood pressure cuff that is user dependent, records a questionable pressure for a split second out of a person's life, and extrapolates that number to have life-altering significance!

Often my patients fall or are sick, are seen by a nurse, or are brought to the emergency room. During those moments their bodies and minds are stressed, and naturally their blood pressure is elevated. But no one seems to recognize the labile nature of pressure in the elderly; pressures can bounce haphazardly within a wide range, soaring with a trauma as minor as the apprehension that occurs while the Velcro cuff expands on their arms. Blood pressure is so variable that it can fluctuate twenty points just during one visit, especially when people get older; we know that there is a lack of correlation between a body's actual blood pressure and what we measure in the office.[15]

After seeing a specialist or coming home from the hospital, many of my elderly patients emerge on more blood pressure medicines than they had going in. And very often, that is when they really start getting sick. The reality is that in the elderly I have seen much more illness caused by low pressure and the medicine used to treat hypertension than from high blood pressure itself, even though the parameters of normal pressure in the elderly are unknown and are probably higher than we think. Simply equating blood pressure reduction to high-quality care, as quality indicators declare, obfuscates the importance in many old bodies of allowing the pressure to climb, at least some of the time. I find it interesting that Medicare's quality indicators focus on preventing modestly high pressures, but say nothing about pushing pressures too low or side effects that occur with antihypertensive medicines.

Recently one of my patients saw a cardiologist, who constantly found her pressure to be very high. He put her on medicines, first one, then two, then five. The pressure did not drop, at least not while she was in his office. She admitted that when his nurse placed the cuff on her arm she became nervous, and that likely caused a spike in pressure. Now she lived in fear of stroke, taking her medicines religiously. But she could hardly stand up. She passed out several times, and became less able to walk. Even with physical therapy, her mobility declined, and she started to sleep more during the day. Her son bought her a blood pressure cuff and instructed her to check the pressure multiple times a day. Instead of attending activities, socializing, and exercising, this once strong woman now stayed in her apartment and took her blood pressure during the times she was not napping, reporting the numbers to her son, worrying about what would become of her. It took a lot of persuasion for me to convince her to drop her blood pressure medicines, especially since my advice contradicted that of the "expert" and of her son, but when she did stop them all, she reclaimed her life, becoming the active person she once was. She stopped checking pressure, and although she convinced herself that she was probably going to get a stroke from her decision, she believed that it was worth the benefit of feeling good.

But was she really going to get a stroke? When I was a medical student the SHEP study altered medical thinking by definitively proving that high systolic blood pressure in the elderly instigates strokes. Many since have criticized that study, showing that systolic blood pressure in the moderate-high range does not elevate stroke risk.[16] More significantly, recent studies have shown that in elders with heart disease, low blood pressure causes as many or more strokes as do high pressures.[17] A VA study of over 600,000 people looking at elderly men with kidney disease, many of whom also have diabetes, showed that lowering blood pressure below 130 led to increased death and no improvement in kidney function. As with studies that look at pressures in older people with strokes and heart attacks, this study found the optimal systolic blood pressure to be 130–160,[18] which is far higher a number than most doctors, patients, and Medicare feel is acceptable.

Still, we in the medical world became obsessed with SHEP, and despite the very small absolute risk reduction of lowering blood pressure in our elderly patients, and despite the often debilitating side effects and interactions from pharmaceutical treatments, we push medicines and check more labs, as the quality indicators compel us to do. What is not often said about SHEP is that it showed marginal increased frequency of stroke only with systolic blood pressure above 160. And yet clinical indicators insist we address blood pressure in the elderly if they are above 120, despite no conclusive evidence that any redution below 160 confers benefit.

One study, SPRINT, small and unpublished but widely reported in the press, has suggested that there are medical benefits of lowering systolic blood pressure in elders below 120. One investigator, Dr. Paul Whelton, said that "there seems to be very convincing evidence of dramatic benefit" of lowering blood pressure below 120 by adding on an additional drug.[19] But there were few participants over the age of seventy, participants all had heart disease and were heavily screened, and the benefits of the add-on drugs likely were independent of their blood pressure lowering properties. These drugs (beta blockers and ace inhibitors) can reduce death in people with congestive heart failure and ischemic heart disease regardless of the blood pressure reduction they induce. In fact, regardless of whether SPRINT's reduction in death was related to lowering blood pressure or from benefiting heart disease, the results were hardly as impressive as the press and trial investigators proclaim. There were 3.5 fewer deaths a year out of 1,000 who lowered their blood pressure below 120 compared to 1,000 who maintained higher pressure (in other words, 997 out of 1,000 people did not benefit), and there were 12 additional severe side effects out of 1,000 in the aggressive blood pressure reduction group compared to the baseline group. As to how many people in the aggressively treated group fell, were dizzy, tired, more confused, and felt worse is not something that this trial addresses. Clearly the bulk of evidence suggests aggressive treatment of blood pressure in the elderly is not beneficial and may be harmful. The SPRINT trial of nine thousand people does not overturn the collective trials of over a million people that demonstrate the danger of aggressive blood pressure control.

We do know that lowering pressures below 120 can cause major complications and side effects, even though doctors who push pressures down below that level are lauded for adhering to quality indicators. Many of my patients are more energetic and cognitively alert at higher pressures, and many of my patients with poor balance fall less often and walk better when their pressure medicines are reduced. Likely their bodies are smarter than we are. (And they haven't read Medicare's quality indicators!) Predictably, pushing blood pressure too low causes cognitive decline, fatigue, and worse balance. When doctors use medicine to reduce pressure below even 130, studies show that there is a potential for causing harm, including an increased death rate and more heart attacks and strokes.[20] A 2015 study also shows that elders receiving aggressive blood pressure treatment have more falls and cardiovascular events.[21] Some studies have shown that the withdrawal of blood pressure medicines typically causes no meaningful elevation of pressure or induction of cardiovascular disease in the majority of the elderly.[22] Given that we have no evidence that pushing blood pressure below 160 is beneficial to the elderly, and that we do have evidence that pushing blood pressure below 120 may be harmful and debilitating to the elderly, it seems that Medicare's quality indicators actually encourage doctors to practice in a way that is more likely to be dangerous than helpful.

More significantly, the drugs used to treat high blood pressure all have significant side effects and interactions that are accentuated as additional drugs are tossed into an older body. Many of my patients are more tired, confused, and dizzy on their blood pressure medicine, and such medicines are more likely to cause falls and fractures.[23] I have seen people hospitalized, incapacitated, and killed by these drugs. Still, many of my patients, families, and doctors would rather obtain a perfect blood pressure number, despite what little it will do for the patient's actual health, rather than worry about how the drugs used to achieve that result may cause some minor "inconveniences" that incapacitate and maim them. Fixing the number has become a compulsion in our medical community, although it is an illusion built on the backs of our patients' health.

Diabetes

Medicare Quality Indicators state that in diabetics between 18–75 A1C should be maintained under 8, LDL cholesterol kept under 100, and blood pressure under 140/90. Presumably all these abnormal numbers are expected to be fixed with medicines. The guidelines also recommend periodic kidney, eye, and foot exams.[24]

Diabetes is another disease where the number is everything. People with type 2 diabetes, or who are considered at risk for it, are frequently asking me to check their sugar, and often they check it on their own, multiple times a day, pricking their fingers to obtain a number they assign too much meaning to, a number that, if too high for example, even transiently, may portend devastating consequences. We are so obsessed with diabetes in our society that we have lowered the threshold of what it means to be diabetic, and have even invented the term "prediabetes" to demonstrate that even slightly high blood sugars could be a sign of trouble ahead. We watch sugars closely, measure another number called A1C that gives us an average sugar over three months, and stress over whether we have achieved ideal diabetic control. Medicare's quality guidelines are somewhat forward thinking in not mandating tight control of type 2 diabetes in patients over the age of seventy-five, but they also do nothing to dissuade that practice. In fact Medicare pays for test strips, blood tests, and specialist visits for even the oldest diabetics and does not comment on whether aggressively controlling sugars is efficacious for everyone. We as doctors are downgraded by the quality indicators for allowing sugars to drift too high in diabetics under seventy-five, but we are not chastised for overtreating sugars with insulin and pills, something that is frankly dangerous and potentially deadly. While treating diabetes in a sensible way is reasonable, simply focusing on the numbers and applauding when they are very low can be clinically deceptive.

The reality is that in the elderly, there is scant evidence that maintaining tight control of blood sugars will confer any benefit at all. In fact, recent studies suggest just the opposite: controlling sugars strictly will actually trigger worse outcomes, including causing *more* death and *more* disability.[25] My own patients are adversely impacted when their sugars drop too low; not only can low sugar immediately kill them, but when they walk around with low sugars they are tired, dizzy, and confused, in a way similar to my patients who have low blood pressure.[26] In nursing home–eligible patients, in fact, a 2012 study showed improved function and fewer deaths in diabetics with the *worst* sugar control (A1C between eight and nine).[27] Like with many hypertensives, diabetics work diligently to normalize their numbers and push them as low as possible even though such aggressive number normalization exposes them to harm and deterioration in quality of life. *The lower the better* seems to be the mantra in our diabetic universe. The number itself seems to obscure what aggressively fixing the number actually is doing to our patients.

Recently one of my patients, who is over ninety and living alone, although plagued by many chronic problems including pain, oxygen-dependent lung disease, and poor balance, saw her endocrinologist. The doctor was not happy with her blood sugar control; her A1C had drifted over eight, and her twice-a-day sugar checks were sometimes close to 200 (something that occurred primarily after she ate). Although she was already on pills, the endocrinologist started insulin, persuading my patient that she had to start injecting herself with needles. My patient was very concerned about her sugars and believed that her life was in jeopardy if they remained elevated. When she started the insulin, her A1C came down to 7.3, although sugars occasionally dropped below eighty, something that made her happy, but frightened me. I explained that she would gain no clinical ground by lowering sugar further; there would not be any reduced risk of stroke, heart attack, kidney disease, death, and so on. If anything, she may hurt herself. But my patient was not moved by my reasoning. She wanted low numbers. Nothing else seemed to matter.

When I am evaluated by quality indicators, there is an assumption that I will use medicines to fix people's sugars when they drift too high. But how good are diabetic medicines? Certainly they are very effective at lowering sugars and A1C. If that were our endpoint of therapeutic success (as it is in the guidelines), then they would be wonderful treatments. But most of them have multiple interactions and side effects and, in some cases, have been shown to actually increase the chances of instigating a major medical event such as a heart attack and death.[28] Still, even after knowing this, many of my patients or their caregivers prefer relying on medicines over allowing numbers to escalate beyond what they have been told is normal. Often my patients' families are the cause of this behavior. Just today an older man with very mild dementia told me his son calls him every morning to ensure that dad checks his sugars. "I just make up numbers," the man said to me. "I give my son sugars that make him happy. I haven't really checked my sugars for months; I just throw out the supplies when they come. But I don't want him upset with me." Although the man believed he was being negligent, in fact he was taking a more prudent path than his son, or society, encouraged of him. He felt well, he was not stressed by his numbers, and likely he would live longer and better than had he been more diligent with his glucose control. He may have failed Medicare's quality indicators, but he was receiving quality care.

Cholesterol

Medicare Quality Indicators look at the need to check and reduce LDL cholesterol in certain conditions such as hypertension, diabetes, and coronary artery disease. They use LDL of 100 above which is abnormal, but do not comment on how to treat.[29]

Number fixation is perhaps most evident in the realm of cholesterol. I have had patients who want to know their cholesterol simply so they can talk about it at dinner with their friends. I have families who fear taking their mom or dad off cholesterol medicine even though they are dementia patients confined to a nursing home, so fearful are they that the cholesterol number will worsen when off the medicines. Cholesterol is easy to measure, is in the news, and has entered our common lore as being a marker of how healthy we are. By fixing cholesterol we are cheating death.

One of my patients came to me on two cholesterol medicines and a few supplements that also control cholesterol. Looking through his records I could find no good diagnoses that would support such aggressive treatment (no heart disease, no strokes, etc.), and his last cholesterol check was perfect. I advised him to eliminate one of his medicines, Zetia, which has been shown to lower cholesterol numbers without significantly lowering rates of heart attacks or strokes.[30] He reluctantly agreed, but several months later, when he asked me to recheck his cholesterol, his numbers had gone up. He became very nervous.

"These labs are not good," he said to me. "I don't want to walk around with those cholesterol levels."

I tried to reassure him. "The numbers may not be perfect," I said, "but they're OK. And stopping the Zetia hasn't increased your risk of getting any illness. You are just on one less medicine, that's all."

He accepted my explanation, for a day or two. But the next week he called my office and asked for a refill of his Zetia. He simply could not bear to live with the higher numbers, even if fixing those numbers did nothing to improve his chance of living better or longer. The illusion of perfect numbers was more important to him than the reality of what those numbers really meant.

There is great controversy about whether any treatment of cholesterol in the elderly is warranted.[31] Statins have been shown to help people with heart disease and strokes, but recent evidence has shown minimal clinically significant benefit in elderly people without risk factors.[32] Even the studies that claim some improvement in outcome among selected elders on statins show a tiny absolute risk reduction usually measured in days of life saved. Cholesterol medicines have significant side effects in the elderly, especially muscle weakness and pain, and do have interactions with other medicines.

They can impair quality of life and they add another element of stress to an older person's already stressful life.

One can argue, despite the conflicting evidence, that after a stroke or heart attack, or even in patients at high risk for such events, statin drugs are potentially efficacious if patients have a reasonably long life expectancy. But that is true despite their cholesterol number. The fact that Zetia can drop the cholesterol number as much as a statin, but that only the latter actually meaningfully reduces reoccurrence of stroke or heart attack in certain people, implies that the number alone is not what is really important. Many doctors try to push that number as low as possible by adding more and more medicines, believing that the number itself has singular significance; up until recently they were supported by clinical guidelines that compelled them to view LDL as a marker of disease. Interestingly, new guidelines actually dissuade doctors from reducing LDL to a predefined target value.[33] That is a breath of fresh air in our number-obsessed medical world; the guidelines actually suggest the use of statins in specific clinical situations where patients may benefit, regardless of their cholesterol numbers, and with attention paid to their age. Cholesterol is just a number. Patients are much more complicated than numbers.

Osteoporosis and More

Medicare Quality Indicators suggest that all people over the age of sixty-five should be screened for osteoporosis by bone density testing, and that people over the age of fifty with known osteoporosis should be prescribed medicines for their condition.[34]

Many of our treatments and guidelines are based on negligible absolute risk reduction and poor data that are not applicable to most elderly patients, while inducing side effect and interaction profiles that put old patients at risk for functional decline, impaired quality of life, and serious medical complications. Examples include osteoporosis medicines like alendronate (Fosamax) that can improve poor bone density numbers (T scores) when evaluated by bone densitometry testing, but that may have marginal to negligible absolute benefit on fracture risk, which is a much more clinically relevant endpoint. While studies tout a 55 percent relative reduction of hip fracture risk for women who use bisphosphonates like alendronate, the absolute risk reduction is much smaller, such that for every thousand women in the high osteoporotic risk group who take alendronate, approximately two will have hip fractures prevented. While the drugs do seem to have more efficacy in preventing spine fractures, those fractures are often found on X-rays but do not cause any pain, and thus are not clinically significant.[35] Certainly there is little or no evidence that alendronate helps prevent hip fractures in lower-risk women without prior fracture, and it has a negligible impact on spine fracture in this group.[36] Bisphosphonates also have multiple common side effects, such as increased bone pain and worse acid reflux. Recent studies suggest that long-term use of alendronate can actually cause increased risk of spontaneous fractures, causing some to advocate limiting their use to five years.[37] Thus we can fix numbers with bisphosphonates, we can demonstrate impressive relative risk improvements, but in fact the drug will help two high-risk women prevent fractures in a year for every thousand women who must take it on a regular basis and expose themselves to drug interactions and medical risk. It can also increase fracture risk with long-term use. Measuring and fixing a bone density number has nebulous clinical value.

Measuring and tightly controlling thyroid disease, anemia, testosterone deficiency, kidney failure, and various other abnormal numbers that can be discovered through tests and "improved" by medicine can be similarly ineffective if not harmful. Mild thyroid disease, for example, rarely causes meaningful clinical improvement when treated with replacement, and yet such treatment and number fixing is considered the standard of care in geriatrics. Anemia is common in the elderly, frequently looked for by a blood test, sometimes treated (typically with iron, which can constipate people), but rarely does treatment lead to clinically meaningful outcomes unless the condition is severe. We are told to measure and fix vitamin levels, monitor kidney and liver function regularly, check urine for blood and protein, check heights and weights and pressures at every visit. So many numbers translate to so many diagnoses that lead to so many medicines, with so little evidence that our deluge of probing and treating is truly helping our older patients live longer and better. And when you add up all the medicines that one of my patients may require to repair his aberrant numbers, the side effects and interactions multiply. The medical community's fixation on numbers, and the recent push to equate number fixing with quality care, has become more important than the reality of what the medicines used to treat those numbers may be actually doing to the patients forced to swallow them.

Treating Annoying Problems in the Aged

On September 11, 2001, at 9:00 a.m., Mrs. M. walked into my office for her appointment. She had a litany of complaints to share with me, and so she whipped out her two-page list.

My memories of 9/11 are infused with Mrs. M.'s visit. It seemed interminable. Between items on her list that ranged from sore toes to bad breath, heads started popping around my exam room door relaying bits of information that were both shocking and unbelievable—a single-engine plane hit the World Trade Center tower, no it turns out it was a commercial jet, the second tower was hit, the Pentagon was hit—and I jolted out of the room and ran down the hall to watch with so many other silent bodies the events that were to transform our world.

"Sorry about that," I would say after every excursion to the TV, as I returned to my visit with Mrs. M. "It looks like there is a full-scale terrorist attack against us."

"Really?" she said. "That is too bad. Well, going down, number 13, I have a small growth on my back I want you to look at."

From that day on, Mrs. M. became Mrs. 9/11. I joked with her about it for many years. She always shook her head, embarrassed, claiming she had not realized what was transpiring that day until she returned to her apartment and turned on the TV. So intent was she in dissecting her list that nothing beyond its twenty-plus issues penetrated her thoughts.

The list is everything to many of my patients. It is imperative at every visit that they recite its contents and that I acknowledge the severity of every one of its items. It took me years of practice to realize that patients like Mrs. 9/11 never expect me to resolve their listed woes, but rather to simply empathize with and recognize the manifestations of aging. Every item on her list, every problem that comes with aging, can be analyzed, tested, and treated. For every ailment there is a test and a medicine, but there rarely is a cure.

With aging comes not only disease but also disability. Nuisance problems crop up like weeds, and often they can impair a person's ability to function independently. From fatigue, to urinary incontinence, to constipation, to various types of pain, aging is not without its challenges. Most elderly people have two choices for how to confront nuisance: try to extirpate it or try to deal with it. The latter is accomplished by means of accommodation and acclimation, and is the recipe for successful aging. The former leads to stress, adverse consequences, tests, excessive medicine use, frustration, and often increased disability.

A variety of drugs exist that erase the ravages of aging, most of them cluttered with potential side effects, few of them able to produce anything but marginal absolute risk reduction. There are incontinence drugs like Ditropan and Detrol, GERD medicines like Nexium and Protonix, erectile dysfunction (ED) medicines like Viagra and Cialis. To many of my patients there is no better way to confront nuisance than with medicines, and for every problem an elderly person can develop there is a drug to fix it. TV ads are cluttered with grateful people having been cured of their enlarged prostates, their incontinence, their erectile dysfunction, their pain. I have never seen such happy people as those who live in the world of TV drug ads. Drug ads cannot tell lies, but they can show only people who improve dramatically, cite only the studies that support them, tell us only the good that is achieved (other than the quickly mumbled list of side effects at the end of every ad that we have become conditioned to ignore).

Americans take more medicines than anyone else in the world, without better outcomes and typically without life-preserving or life-improving results.[38] Those of us who practice geriatric medicine fight every day to get people off their long list of medicines touted to cure practically everything and to be absolutely essential to their health and well-being. It is a battle against a powerful message, one that promises that aging itself can be cured. It is a battle against many deep-seated perceptions, underscored by the quality indicators with which Medicare will now be judging us. When we do win, we almost always see satisfying results. But when we lose, we watch our patients decline, still convinced that all of their fifteen drugs and supplements are necessary, still happy about the thoroughness of their care, but still unable to dance in the woods like those people on the TV commercials.

Dementia

Medicare Quality Indicators recommend various tests for dementia that allow the disease to be characterized and staged, as well as various forms of screening and counseling, but do not comment on the use of medication in its treatment.[39]

Dementia is perhaps the most devastating illness for which patients and families seek a miracle solution. While some of the elderly simply become forgetful, an outcome that is expected as people age, others lapse into true dementia, where function declines and the brain's capacity to reason collapses. Several drugs are promoted as capable of improving dementia, especially Alzheimer's disease, such as Aricept, Exelon, and Namenda. But again, despite curves and graphs that demonstrate the remarkable relative risk reduction of disease progression from these drugs, the absolute clinical improvement is negligible for most patients, while the studies themselves may be unreliable.[40]

No drugs actually alter the course of dementia; at best they help symptoms. Improvement in clinical trials is measured by numbers; patients take a test, typically scored on a scale of seventy, and if they improve their score by four points or more then the drug is believed to be effective. It is unclear how much these research-derived numerical scales actually translate to clinically relevant change. In fact, studies that measure functional improvement that is recognized by their caregivers are less convincing. Most of the time numerical improvement, even with these scales, has been small, and the dropout rate of patients from the studies due to side effects has been very high.[41] Also, none of the studies extend beyond a year in duration, and the improvement that is seen seems to level off after about four to six months, after which drug efficacy parallels placebo.[42] So it is unclear just how long the very modest effect of these drugs will persist. Studies have shown that approximately 9 to 30 percent of people with dementia who take these drugs have some symptomatic improvement compared to placebo.[43] But interestingly, approximately 30 percent of people with dementia have a response to placebo, showing that there is a very large placebo effect to treatment.[44] Namenda, a newer and more expensive drug, has even less evidence to back its use.[45] Also, no study has demonstrated that any one drug is better than another, or that a combination of these drugs is better than a single drug alone.[46] Again, even those who do have a response often have a clinically marginal change for a very brief duration; typically they merely demonstrate a transient improvement in their memory-score numbers.

On the drugs or off, people with dementia decline, become disabled and nonfunctioning, and may eventually require twenty-four-hour care or admission to long-term-care facilities. The drugs offer illusory hope that this terrible disease can somehow be stopped in its tracks. Often they are used as a crutch, while other more proven methods of helping people with dementia are neglected, such as socialization and exercise.[47] The drugs also have substantial side effects. About 10 percent of people on these drugs have significant gastrointestinal side effects that force them to stop the medicines,[48] and a small but measurable number have very serious side effects such as complete heart block, fainting, and hip fractures.[49] Medicare B pays for tests and specialty visits; Medicare D pays for the drugs. No part of Medicare will help patients with dementia or their families pay for day care, home care, exercise programs, or other proven methods of helping them cope with the disease.

Pharmaceutical representatives who have talked to me claim that not only do these drugs help slow the progression of Alzheimer's disease in a significant way (and they have skewed graphs to prove it), but also that if the drug is stopped the patient will lose everything he or she has gained from the drug and will never recover. Such scare tactics convince doctor and patient alike that not using this miracle of science is irresponsible and cruel, and stopping the drug is even worse. Many neurologists and psychologists with whom I work convince patients and families that these drugs are both necessary and effective. Quality indicators and clinical guidelines encourage doctors to treat dementia, and the treatments most available and accepted are these drugs. Such drugs are just another example of how we have all been convinced that aggressive treatment can cure the worst ravages of aging by fixing nebulous numbers, even if such lore diverges far from the truth and can actually be harmful and deceptive.

Drug Advertising

Pharmaceutical companies, often much maligned by those who seek to reform our health-care industry, benefit greatly by our quest to repair numbers and symptoms of aging with medicines. The clinical studies that they sponsor report dramatic medication impact almost exclusively in relative risk/benefit language. That language is then picked up by the press, which reports it to the public. We hear frequently about 50 percent risk reduction, 20 percent improvement, and other often deceiving figures that obscure whether a drug is truly beneficial. The risks of drugs are typically glossed over. In addition, pharmaceutical companies advertise directly to the public, using doctor and patient actors to demonstrate medication wonderment. But perhaps most concerning is how such companies market their drugs to the health-care delivery industry, coaxing doctors and other professionals to believe that the answer to much of aging's decline lies in a bottle of pills.

Many studies have explored the intoxicating impact of drug advertising,[50] and I do not plan to comment extensively on that reality other than saying that many of my elderly patients, and their families, believe that medicines can repair much of what is going wrong with aging because of what they have seen or read in ads. Drug companies have a right to advertise and try to sell their products. It is not their actions that are most disturbing. It is rather the fact that doctors and patients alike buy into their message. It is that the lay press publishes their dogma, using relative risk to demonstrate a drug's magical properties without exploring whether the drug really is clinically efficacious. It is that few even in academic medicine try to counter the myths. The impact of pharmaceutical companies on the medical community is well documented,[51] and I am no more immune to its power than any others.

During my early days as a doctor I appreciated an occasional foray into Baltimore for a good time. Our local drug reps were always happy to accommodate. They invited us out quite frequently, sometimes to restaurants, sometimes to Orioles games, sometimes even on trips. A few of us from work would accept and go as a group. There we would start with an open bar and a bowl of jumbo shrimp, then a brief talk by a doctor paid by the drug company to say something nice about a particular drug under the guise of an unbiased scientific talk, then we would have our full meal with steak and potatoes and dessert. It was something I looked forward to and became almost addicted to after a while. I saw nothing wrong with it. But then one day, after a very mediocre drug dinner at the newly opened ESPN Zone, the drug rep who sponsored the dinner walked into my office and, in front of patients, handed me a trophy as a gesture of thanks for using his drug. To me that was a wake-up call, and my taste for pharmaceutical-sponsored dinners abruptly ended.

When I was a resident at the University of Virginia, where the faculty looked down on drug reps and attempted to keep them out of the institution (even while many of them were being paid by drug companies either to do research or to give talks, something endemic in the world of academic medicine),[52] we welcomed the reps because they provided us with something we needed and, we felt, deserved. Residency was difficult, to say the least, and we were paid very little to work like dogs. The drug reps offered us a package of perks and a few slaps on the back. My favorite rep sold nicotine patches, which at the time were prescription drugs. He financed a program I ran to help patients and employees quit smoking, providing me with free patches to give to my class participants. He twice sent me and twenty other residents on an amazing weekend adventure to the New River Gorge in West Virginia for a white water rafting trip. When I left residency he offered to fly me and my family to Lake Tahoe to participate in a smoking cessation workshop, where we would be wined and dined for a week. He was always good to me, and never seemed to ask for anything in return. Throughout residency various reps provided us with weekly lunches, meals at good Charlottesville restaurants, and even trips to local resorts. In fact, my drug company perks constituted some of the best memories of those three years. Such extravagance is no longer permitted, although one can still find a good lunch or dinner gratis if one looks around any medical corner.

Some drug reps are true salesmen, such as the man who gave me a trophy, but most I have encountered genuinely believe in their drugs and want to convince us to share in that belief. They do not force us to use any particular medicine. It is our choice what we actually prescribe. Sometimes patients request drugs they have seen advertised, sometimes doctors prescribe drugs that drug reps convince them are effective; almost always Medicare D will pay for those choices. But wrapped around every decision to use a medicine is a deep-seated contention that medicines can cure virtually everything, and that newer medicines are even more effective than their predecessors. And the language of all pharmaceutical reps with whom I have had contact is that of relative risk.

One troubling practice of pharmaceutical companies is making sure that their reps fill doctors' closets with free samples of all the newest and most expensive medicines. In my current practice, where I have established no ties with drug companies and thus have no free pens, lunches, or samples, I cannot offer any free boxed medicines to my patients, and several patients have even thought about leaving me because of that. They have become very dependent on the samples, especially when it comes to expensive medicines. Those who have good insurance start with the samples and then buy the medicines, the precise formula that the drug companies count on.[53] Once our patients become accustomed to those drugs, they will in any case need to pay for the medicine, have their insurance pay for it, or become dependent on a supply of samples. Either way, they are now taking a new, expensive medicine while an older, more tested medicine could have been given in its stead, or perhaps no medicine at all.

During one of President Obama's town meetings to promote his Affordable Care Act, a member of the audience who supported health-care reform said indignantly that his insurance company had tried to switch him from brand-name Lipitor to generic simvastatin, and that his heart doctor wanted him on Lipitor, and how would the president's plan prevent such an outrage. I was curious to see how President Obama would respond. In fact, he tried to explain that often a less expensive generic like simvastatin is equally effective and should be the preferred drug. But his statement, which was bravely accurate, seemed to soar over the head of the man, who continued to complain about having to take generics. There are generics for virtually every major drug class that work just as well (or equally not as well, as the case may be) as the more expensive drugs. But no one promotes the generics. No generic drug makers give doctors lunches, provide samples, or flood the market with ads to push their drugs. Prilosec (omeprazole), when it came out, revolutionized treatment of acid reflux. They called it the purple pill, and we were bombarded by advertising proclaiming its revolutionary benefits. But when its patent expired, the parent drug company of omeprazole invented Nexium, the new purple pill. Omeprazole changed its color and became relegated to the status of cheap ineffective generic, while Nexium was the new miracle drug. The ploy worked. Nexium supplanted Prilosec in the hearts and minds of American consumers. Omeprazole became just another generic medicine. Both Omeprazole and Nexium are similarly efficacious and with identical side effects.[54]

In my recent career I have found that many of the products most heavily advertised by pharmaceutical companies are copycat drugs, something borne out by the literature.[55] These are drugs that do not have a novel purpose, but rather tweak an existing drug to give it a new patent and a more expensive price tag. Then the company's scientists work hard to prove that the new drug is somehow superior to the virtually identical medicines already on the market; they bend some curves and exaggerate some relative risk numbers, and then at least for a few years they feed their reps with enough ammo to peddle the drugs to hungry doctors and consumers.

The point is that we already have too many drugs on the market that are of questionable efficacy. These can include "cures" for urinary incontinence, depression, and acid reflux, to name a few. Do incontinence medicines really work? Probably not, but they all can cause their patients to have dry mouth, constipation, more falls, and worse confusion. Acid reflux medicines, though often able to relieve symptoms of heartburn, can increase the risk of bone fractures while providing questionable long-term efficacy. We use many depression medicines to "cure" fatigue and boredom, common problems in the elderly better treated with socialization and exercise, free of the very real side effects most depression medicines deliver.[56] We treat toenail fungus, arthritis, dizziness, poor appetite, drippy noses, constipation, and so many other common ailments in our aging patients with drugs that are nominally effective, interact with other medicines, and have a laundry list of frequent side effects. Drugs cannot cure the ravages of aging. Usually they just get in the way.

Supplements

As a sidenote, I should state that supplements and vitamins are not necessarily any better than prescription pills. They also have side effects and interactions and, unlike medicines, most are not well regulated by the FDA, nor are they well studied. Two miracle drugs that were evaluated for their curative powers in heart disease were folic acid and vitamin E. Both, after they were subjected to good double-blind placebo studies, and despite theoretical promise for their worth, were found to be ineffective and perhaps harmful.[57] A more recent study of vitamin E did show some benefit in people with dementia,[58] but the research on memory supplements is very fickle, and a positive study is often followed by a negative one. Also, the improvements are typically clinically of minimal significance.

Folic acid is not Folate or Folinic acid. Folic acid blocks Folate receptors from uptake of Folate.

People with memory loss also reach for coconut oil and ginseng, despite a complete lack of evidence that any of these or so many other products accomplish anything of value.[59] Calcium supplementation, which is recommended for older people and is widely taken by my patients, has never been demonstrated to definitively reduce fracture rates in older people, *✕* and potentially can increase the risk of heart attacks and other untoward effects.[60] Fish oil, which is also popular among my patients, has not *always* been demonstrated to reduce heart disease, and may have significant side effects such as increasing cancer risk.[61] Aspirin,[62] multiple vitamins, and antioxidants[63] all have been promoted to alleviate the problems that come with aging, but these supplements are often either ineffective or actually harmful. In fact, even more than with pharmaceuticals, supplements can promise the world and deliver nothing, as they are not subject to any rigorous FDA standards. In addition they interact with other medicines and add to a patient's expansive medicine burden within his/her body. Now we hold vitamin D up as a new savior, with a few small studies cited to support its wonderment. Perhaps it will prove to be of use, perhaps not, but certainly it will not reverse the nuisances and disability that inevitably accompany aging. *You still need sunlight exposure!*

One cannot discount the impact of persuasion on the perceived value of a drug or supplement. When friends and doctors and advertisements and TV shows pound into someone's head that a drug is good, then often that person will believe it is working, even if it does nothing at all. Such a phenomenon is called the placebo effect.[64] We have already discussed that 30 percent of people who take a placebo in dementia studies improve their memory scores; such a placebo benefit is common with many drugs we use. A 2015 study showed that approximately 50 percent of people with depression improved when they took placebos, an effect ascribed to the production of cerebral neurochemicals triggered by the positive expectation derived by taking the drug.[65] A study published in 2011 examined the power of placebos when patients with upper respiratory infections received either placebo or the herb echinacea. Those who believed that echinacea works to help colds, and those who thought they were receiving the herb, regardless of whether they received the open-label medicine or a placebo, had a significantly shorter duration of their cold and a less severe cold. Their belief in the herb's power caused them to have clinical improvement.[66]

Vit E studies only used a fraction of the vitamin and didn't include any tocotrienols, etc..

✱ Calcium must be taken with Vit D for uptake and Vit K2 so it ends up in your bones, not your arteries, etc.

With many of our drugs and supplements, the placebo effect may be the most potent benefit patients will receive.* As an intern at the University of Virginia Hospital I worked under a resident who was a bit odd. He could not tolerate patients, many of whom were admitted to the hospital every week, who came in with complaints of vague pain and then demanded narcotics. One night he assembled us and a few willing nurses to take care of an infamous pain-medication seeker. He told the patient that he had access to a new drug, Norsaline, which was stronger than any other pain reliever available, but that it could wreak havoc on the body and needed to be monitored closely. Would the patient want to try it? The patient, who was writhing in pain, agreed. We put him in a room and hooked him up to an IV, as several nurses monitored his vital signs. Then the resident started the "Norsaline drip," which was in fact a bag of saline, or salt water. Nurses shouted out vital signs with theatrical consternation, the resident changed the rate of flow, chaos consumed the room. After the bag finished, the patient smiled, saying he never felt better in his life.

That is the power of placebo, an impact imparted by so many of our drugs and supplements, and by so much of our medical delivery system. Normal saline of course was safe, even if the ethics of the resident's actions could be questioned. But many of the other drugs we prescribe for our elderly patients are not so innocuous, even if they often do offer a very valuable placebo benefit. Given the harsh impact of drugs on the elderly, and the costs of such treatment, our promotion of drugs as an answer to aging's woes is a dangerous seed to plant. *AMEN!*

Clinical Guidelines

We have talked about clinical guidelines largely in the context of Medicare's quality indicators. Clinical guidelines are consensus statements drafted by "experts" in a particular field largely based on the conclusions of prevailing medical literature. They are typically extremely generic; it is rare that guidelines are applicable to elderly patients whose multiple illnesses, medicines, expectations, susceptibility to side effects, and life expectancy make each older person unique and not able to be squeezed into the rigid mold of a guideline. Also, as discussed, many studies used to script guidelines are sponsored by pharmaceutical companies and evaluate few

check out "nocebo effect" to blow your mind

elderly subjects. And many of their "expert" authors have questionable motives, a specialized agenda, and minimal understanding of the aging process.[67] A 2014 *Annals of Internal Medicine* editorial suggested that clinical guidelines do have some validity, but while primary-care doctors like me disdain the highly interventional guidelines scripted by specialists, the specialists similarly scoff at the anti-interventional guidelines developed in the academic primary-care community. All guidelines, the author suggests, are sensationalized by the press in a way that obscures their real value.[68] Guidelines also will fluctuate based on which group pens them, and in what year they are penned. Some guidelines from the last decade would be considered substandard medical care today. If we are going to place clinical guidelines on a pedestal and label them an effective foundation on which to base quality medical care, then we have to admit that many doctors have practiced, and continue to practice, poor medical care by adhering to guidelines that have been discredited, and that perhaps the doctors of tomorrow will disparage us for adhering to the soon-to-be discredited guidelines of today.

Medicare's quality indicators are fairly basic guidelines with some flexibility built into them. Many are based on the US Preventive Services Task Force (USPSTF) guidelines that tend to be very conservative in their recommendations. But the quality indicators stress when to test and treat, rather than when not to. They are also far too generic to be relevant to many of the older patients we are being instructed to use them on. And to many of us in primary care, quality indicators force us to devote too much of our effort to documenting how often we order certain tests, fix certain numbers, and use certain medicines by employing a tightly scripted format that is time consuming and not constructive, rather than discussing medical issues with our patients and allowing them to participate in the decision-making progress.

In some larger health plans physicians are judged by specific clinical guidelines, many of which encourage them to fix the very numbers that we have demonstrated have little relevance to the elderly, such as tight control of hypertension and diabetes, and the use of statins in patients with high cholesterol.[69] Two of the primary innovations of Medicare reform and the ACA—the development of accountable care organizations (ACOs) and of quality indicators called PQRS (both of which we will talk about in more detail later)—presume that patient outcome can be improved by adherence to specified clinical guidelines, and that such adherence can be used to define a physician's performance. In the northern Maryland ACO to which I have been assigned, I will be judged by how well I control sugars, blood pressure, and cholesterol and how often I prescribe specific types of drugs that are deemed to be efficacious in conditions such as congestive heart failure and coronary artery disease.[70] Clinical guidelines are becoming a vital instrument used to drive health-care reform; gradually a larger part of our Medicare payment is becoming contingent on our compliance with the quality indicators. Pay for performance is being touted as an effective way to cut costs and improve quality.

But how effective are mandated performance measures that are scripted from clinical guidelines in achieving these goals? It is hard to imagine how asking us to fill out complicated forms indicating how we measure, record, and treat specific ailments and numbers in our elderly patients will save Medicare money. If anything it will lead to more tests, more referrals, more medication use, and more side effects, all at a higher cost. The process of completing ACO and PQRS quality measurement forms, on top of several other "Medicare innovations" that are measuring the "quality" of our care, is laborious and expensive, and takes time away from quality patient discourse. By dictating what we should be discussing with our patients, and by specifically telling us how to have that conversation, quality indicators directly infringe on the doctor-patient relationship. Geriatric medicine is a much more nuanced field than can be measured by preordained quality indicators. My eighty-five-year-old patient in a nursing home and my eighty-five-year-old patient who just came off the golf course have different values, problems, and needs that will impact how they perceive a certain test or intervention. A meaningful discussion between a patient and doctor will lead to a meaningful resolution. None of this can be accomplished within the narrow scope of quality indicators.

Clinical guidelines, by advocating number chasing and treatment, also can lead to polypharmacy, a true danger in the geriatric population. Currently I am recertifying for the internal medicine boards and am taking a home-study course to get myself ready. The tapes I am listening to, fifty hours in all, are copied from a board review course taught by physicians from a major medical center. These people are academics and specialists, picked as being experts in their field, similar to the people who write clinical guidelines and orchestrate Medicare reform. What is most amazing to me is what each of them perceives to be the standard of care in terms of medicine use. The cardiologists would have the vast majority of my elderly patients on between five and ten drugs depending on their conditions, the osteoporosis expert wants at least three drugs and vitamins, the renal doctor is expecting a few drugs and vitamins, the ophthalmologist a few vitamins, and every other specialist a few more drugs, each one said to be absolutely necessary for the survival of that particular specialist's organ of interest. They all demand fairly regular lab testing and number monitoring. What one specialist considers standard of care for a certain ailment another specialist bashes as being harmful to another ailment that is likely to coexist with the first. During the Internal Medicine Boards Review course, one of the cardiologists told us that in congestive heart failure (CHF), a condition that occurs when the heart is not able to capably pump all of its contents to the body, it was standard of care to use certain drugs to adequately treat the condition. Medicare's quality indicators list some, but not all, of the drugs she deemed essential. But then the cardiologist said something both illuminating and frightening. She said that sometimes these essential drugs can cause the blood pressure to drop too low. Don't worry about it, she callously stated. Even if the pressure drops too low, the drugs will still do their job. You just have to be tough and hold your ground.

We as geriatricians know that when the blood pressure is too low our older patients are tired, they fall down and break bones, they are dizzy and confused, and they feel lousy. Maybe they even become sicker and die like the Virginia farmer I treated. So is it really worth it to be on a preordained assortment of drugs and to fix a predefined set of numbers, with perhaps a tiny absolute risk reduction, if the consequences can be functionally disastrous and the outcome not meaningfully improved? And what if the patients are on other drugs for other conditions that interfere with these drugs, or what if these drugs make other conditions they have worse? What is the proof that the four essential drugs for congestive heart failure genuinely help an eighty-five-year-old woman with poor balance, chronic back pain, memory loss, and dizziness who is on eight other medicines? Have studies been conducted that prove efficacy for that patient? The answer is no. The answer is that clinical guidelines, and the vast majority of studies, do not apply to most of my patients.

It is important to understand that there is ample evidence that the more pharmaceutical drugs there are in a person's body, the less effective and more potentially dangerous each drug is, especially as people age.[71] Some have said that when a person is on more than six drugs (including supplements) then the side effects of each one doubles. And some data suggest that up to 400,000 people are killed or maimed every year by adverse drug reactions.[72] Such reactions include organ damage, severe allergies, delirium, and even death. So although each and every drug seems to be necessary to erase and reduce disease burden, fix a number, or improve a nuisance, in combination they can tear an elderly body to shreds. Thus when clinical guidelines push us to measure and fix more numbers, when each number and each nuisance demands more and more drugs for its resolution, a body that sits in delicate balance between function and disarray gets pushed closer to the latter. All of us who practice geriatrics see this happen. But as geriatric doctors, our "performance" will now be measured by our ability to "fix" numbers and flood our patients with even more poison. This is touted as Medicare reform!

Quality indicators, and our fixation with number measurement and number repair through medicines, has led us down a precarious road. Once we believe that an older person's health status can be equated to a number, and once we convince ourselves that by fixing that number with medicines we are fixing the patient, then we are led to believe that aging itself can be fended off by medical science as long as we probe and treat aggressively enough. This is what I label "thorough" medical care. Often my patients, or their families, laud *thorough* doctors who are monitoring their kidney function, or fixing their diabetes, or keeping a tight watch on their heart. Thorough medicine is not necessarily effective medicine; for elderly patients it often causes more harm than good; it raises expectations beyond what is reasonable for doctor and patient alike, and its huge price tag is largely financed by Medicare. But once the idea percolates that aging can be reversed, then a cascade of interventions are possible, each more expensive and potentially dangerous than the next. And so we move down a road of aggressive care, a road flooded with pills of every color and shape, tests of every form, treatments of every type. In a world of common sense, people age, and that is OK. Problems occur that are not amenable to simple fixes, and that is OK, too. We should accept it, and try to promote happiness and activity as age chips away at our patients. We should utilize tests and treatments judiciously, realizing that too much of anything is potentially harmful and that what works for one patient may not work for all. And we should be realistic about the fact that excessive treatment may lead to excessive decline. But in the world today, number chasing and medication obsession are the first ingredients of "thorough" medical care, the dangerous philosophy we will explore throughout the book.

2

Defining Thorough

Finding and Fixing Everything

When a lot of remedies are suggested for a disease,
that means it cannot be cured.

Anton Chekhov

Americans perceive that our current high-tech medical system is the best in the world, despite dubious evidence to support that claim.[1] From MRIs to cardiac stress tests, mammograms to colonoscopies, full blood tests to full exams, we as doctors have at our disposal multiple tools to get inside our patients' bodies and search for trouble.

Technology in health care has skyrocketed in this country. Both doctors and patients are enamored of technology, believing that tests and procedures help eradicate disease and extend life.[2] The use of radiologic imaging in particular is accelerating rapidly without any evidence that X-rays and scans are extending or improving health for the population as a whole.[3] Since the early 1990s the ordering of head CT scans has doubled, chest CT scans have quintupled, head MRIs quadrupled, spine MRIs have increased sixfold, and hip and knee MRIs have increased tenfold.[4] The same is true of procedures touted as lifesaving and that are similarly skyrocketing in their frequency of being performed, despite specious evidence. Says one author who has studied medical care: "Many doctors are happy to embrace the data that confirm their preconceived notions about the effectiveness of invasive treatment, while ignoring studies that don't."[5]

Our oldest patients are afflicted with disease, much of it hidden beneath a thin veil of accommodation. If we look hard enough, we will likely uncover medical conditions that if left alone will never cause harm. Tests allow us to look for and find hidden illness, even if the discovery itself may lead patients down a dangerous road. Tests also produce false-positive results, sometimes at an astonishingly high rate, leading to unnecessary additional tests, procedures, or treatments that may cause patients substantial harm at an extraordinary cost just to prove that the original test was erroneous. But a thorough doctor will look. A thorough doctor will find. And then a thorough doctor will treat. Many studies have been conducted and books written documenting the futility of excessive testing.[6] But a thorough doctor is not discouraged by the negative perceptions portrayed by doubters. If there are medical problems present, despite a patient's age, and despite minimal evidence to support aggressive treatment, we as doctors tend to find those problems and fix them. This is a path that Medicare endorses, as it will pay for tests and procedures more readily than it pays for much else. Medicare pays for diabetics to check their sugars regularly, to see a plethora of specialists, to have surgical procedures to repair the consequences of bad habits, but it will not pay for ongoing nutrition counseling or exercise programs, which would help significantly more at a much lower cost. This is a path that current Medicare reform efforts do little to discourage.

For doctors, following the route of thorough medicine by ordering a lot of tests is the path of least resistance. Nothing is more difficult than trying to explain and reason through the natural declines inherent to aging, than trying to convince patients and their families in this age of scientific marvel trumpeted by the media and the medical community that a minimalist approach is most sensible, than spending excessive time on the phone or in the office discussing something that can be served to them with far less effort and at a far lower cost for them (if a much higher cost for the system) by writing prescriptions and ordering tests. Especially as our office visits are dominated by typing scripted notes on computers and documenting our adherence to clinical guidelines, such discussions become virtually impossible to have.

The "thorough" approach to medical care makes people happy because they think we really care about them. It makes us happy, because we have to spend less time with our patients (since we just write prescriptions for tests and specialist visits and send them on their merry way), and thus can see more patients, giving us more revenue. Lawyers don't sue thorough doctors, families don't yell at thorough doctors, and Medicare rewards thorough doctors by paying them well for their tests and procedures.

No one can deny that aging is a process of incessant decline. For reasons none of us fully comprehend, every part of the body deteriorates simultaneously as people reach advanced age, and even a person who seems to be completely together is really a patchwork of Band-Aids and broken machinery that can be unraveled by one minor insult. I have seen apparently healthy elderly people go from being independent and active members of society to nursing home–dependent skeletons in a matter of weeks without any good scientific explanation as to what exactly precipitated the plunge, and without it slowing despite tens of thousands of dollars of intervention. Such a reality frustrates patients and their families. It does not fit well into the neatly packed narrative that American medical lore has painted for them. There needs to be a reason; things don't just happen. Somewhere out there exists a doctor, test, or procedure that can make sense of an older person's decline and fix it. The more we look for problems, the better chance we have of resolving them. Why give up when there is an answer out there waiting for us, if only we keep plugging at it?

Screening: Prostate Cancer

Mr. L. came to my office for a routine visit. A healthy man in his late eighties, he was independent and vibrant, even if he had slowed down a bit in the last few years. But that did not bother him. He still saw friends and family, took naps when he was tired, did a little reading when his eyes allowed it, and had found a good cocktail of juices and stool softeners to get his bowels moving just about right.

On the day of the visit we both agreed that he had not had a complete exam for a while, so we did one, although I must say that none of us physicians really know what a complete exam is, and there is little evidence that a "complete exam" is of any validity.[7] But as part of this exam I inserted my lubed finger into his rectum, and there I found a surprise. Mr. L.'s prostate was huge and rock hard.

"Are you peeing OK?" I asked him.

"Sure, every day like clockwork. Sometimes I get up at night, but I go right back to sleep."

I explained to Mr. L. the significance of my finding. Very often large, hard prostates indicate prostate cancer. We could get a PSA (prostate-specific antigen) blood test to help confirm it, or I could send him directly to a urologist for a biopsy. Or we could do nothing.

"What would you do?' he asked me, hardly concerned about the potential gravity of what I had just relayed to him.

So I laid out the arguments pro and con. On the one hand, even if he had prostate cancer, it would likely not kill him at his age, and a biopsy was not without risks. On the other hand, if he did have prostate cancer, it could be treated, although there was no real evidence that treatment would lead to a longer or better life, and treatment had its own risks. "If you want," I said, picking some vague middle road, "we can just get the PSA and see what it is before we make a decision. But it's probably going to be high, and it won't change what we do."

"Then," he said with a smile, "let's not do anything for now. If I have problems with my pee, I'll let you know." After all, he told me, he was pretty old. I promised him that I would keep my fingers away from his prostate from now on.

A few years passed, and Mr. L. meandered down to the office one morning complaining that for the past twelve hours he'd been unable to urinate. He felt well, but was just concerned. I was rounding in the hospital, and no other doctors could see him in the office, so the front staff made an urgent appointment with a local urologist. It turned out that by the time he arrived there he was able to pass urine; likely he was a bit dehydrated. But the urologist checked a PSA, as they always do, and the result was an astonishing 150. Now, those of you who understand PSAs know that anything over four is high, over ten is likely cancer, and the highest I had ever seen was about sixty. One hundred fifty is beyond conception.

The urologist did some tests and suggested immediate treatment for what he called aggressive prostate cancer, although Mr. L. had no symptoms. He ordered a hormone injection of a medicine called Lupron that curbs the spread of prostate cancer, which Mr. L. agreed to take. Soon after that injection, Mr. L. became profoundly weak. I saw him and could not ascertain a cause. But he deteriorated quickly, and soon we had to put him in the nursing home temporarily to get him stronger.

Mr. L. was almost ninety when that occurred, healthy as can be. He never left the nursing home, and died somewhere close to his hundredth birthday. He also never walked again. He declined further treatment for his prostate cancer, and clearly that cancer did not kill him. Nor did the cancer cause him any harm. It was the treatment for a harmless cancer that did him in. And his story is more common than people seem to realize.

Tests are potentially dangerous because they lead to unnecessary treatments that can be toxic. The testing process itself—whether a needle or an X-ray—can cause direct harm to the body and send a frail person into a tailspin. Disease, if left alone, can often coexist with an elderly body. Even cancer may not kill many elderly people; some cancers even regress on their own.[8] A large amount of men die with prostate cancer but not of it.[9] The introduction of PSA screening, followed by invasive testing and aggressive treatments for prostate cancer, has not reduced mortality in the elderly.[10] Many people have breast cancer, skin cancers, even colon cancer, and they die of something completely different. Unfortunately, we do not know who may benefit from screening and who may be harmed by it. We can never know. But as people age, the prospect of finding a problem that can save or improve their lives becomes less realistic, while the prospect of causing injury becomes more common.

I talked earlier in the book about a woman who insisted on having PSA measured in her dad. When the PSA was elevated she brought him to a major medical center under the care of experts who continued to test and measure, treat him, and monitor the treatment. His life became consumed by this, to the point where he physically declined from a deluge of stress. That story evokes two very important points. One is that stress can be a salient result of too much testing.[11] When screening tests reveal problems, then a patient has to live with the reality that some horrible process is ravaging his or her body. That pestering thought is very toxic, and it takes the life out of many of my patients. This is not something easy to measure, but it is a reality I see regularly. The second point is that the testing and treatment process can instigate a substantial decline in quality of life, especially after a prostate cancer diagnosis.[12] A British study showed that most men who were retrospectively aware of the implications of their prostate screening regret ever getting it.[13]

When to Screen: The Case of Mammography

In the population at large, finding problems and treating them does not necessarily extend life. Not only do treatments for certain conditions in the elderly such as prostate cancer, breast cancer, pancreatic cancer, lung cancer, and so on, not definitively help reduce mortality, but even more revealing is that many people who are treated for these diseases and "cured" tend to die at the same time they would have even if they had never been tested and treated.[14]

Many organizations, such as the US Preventive Services Task Force (USPSTF), elucidate the utility of screening tests at certain ages. Procedures such as mammograms, PSA tests, and colonoscopies are all given age ranges when they are no longer effective in preventing illness.[15] For most screening tests, it has been shown that utility diminishes and harm increases by age seventy-five. Still, despite this reality, Medicare will continue to pay for those tests as well as for the treatment warranted by what the tests reveal, whether the treatment is deemed useful or not. CMS has talked about paying only for screening tests approved by the US Preventive Services Task Force, but I doubt that will occur in our current politically charged medical environment, where patient demand for "thorough" care often trumps common sense and when rationing of care has become such a dirty word. The case of mammograms is illustrative of my skepticism. An excellent book that demonstrates the discord between the medical utility of mammograms and the hype surrounding their use is Gayle Sulik's *Pink Ribbon Blues*. It reveals a truth that is often obscured by our medical lore about what constitutes thorough care.

Several decades ago CMS changed its rules and permitted mammograms only every other year for older women, a decision supported by copious data. But immediately, protests by women's and consumer groups caused CMS to buckle and revert to the status quo of paying for annual exams at every age. Many researchers question whether the elderly should have mammograms at all. A recent *New England Journal of Medicine* study concluded that most tumors detected by mammograms are not clinically relevant and require no treatment. The study found that 1.3 million women were overdiagnosed in the past thirty years. One thousand women are screened to prevent one breast cancer death, while the screening triggers sixty-three unnecessary biopsies and no proven decrease in overall death.[16] Several other studies similarly cast doubt on mammography as a means of reducing death in the elderly, most notably two by Welch's group at Dartmouth.[17] The most recent study followed 90,000 women for twenty-five years and found no reduction in breast cancer death among women with mammograms compared to those who did not receive mammograms. In addition, because mammograms pick up cancers so early, and since many cancers either grow slowly, do not grow at all, or even regress, the early detection of cancer led to unnecessary surgery, radiation, or even chemotherapy for nonlethal cancers in 2.36 out of 1000 women who received mammograms.[18] A recent op-ed by Welch highlights the uncertainly of screening, pointing to the need for further study to obtain better answers. He cites that among a thousand fifty-year-old US women screened annually for a decade, 0.3 to 3.2 will avoid a breast cancer death, 490 to 670 will have at least one false alarm, and between three and fourteen will have unnecessary treatment. He also notes that many women may not want to be screened if better informed of those numbers.[19] His article was immediately assailed by several physicians, including Barbara Monsees, who chairs the Breast Imaging Commission of the American College of Radiology, and Murray Rebner, president of the Society of Breast Imaging. These authors use relative risk to dramatize the same numbers used by Dr. Welch, stating that "women who get mammograms regularly have a 30 to 45 percent lower risk of dying from breast cancer." They also falsely state that annual mammography is universally endorsed for all women over the age of forty.[20] Clearly, numbers can look dramatic when related as relative risk percentages. In our oldest patients, even the prospect of saving lives is very dubious, and the prospect of causing harm escalates.

No one has demonstrated any significant advantage of screening women over seventy-five years old, who comprise the bulk of my patients. States the USPSTF website: "Among women 75yrs or older, evidence of benefits of mammography is lacking." A 2001 discussion of screening in the elderly suggests that most organizations do recommend that there be an upper age limit to mammography, citing more generally that "some of the greatest harms of screening occur by detecting cancers that would never have been clinically significant. This becomes more likely as life expectancy decreases."[21] An earlier study finds that the prevalence of detecting clinically significant breast cancer through mammography declines with age, citing the potential harm from finding and treating lesions that will not impact mortality.[22] Some of my older patients ask me what the harm is in getting a mammogram: Why not get the test and acquire some information? But there *is* potential for harm. Biopsies are not without risk. Treatments for nonlethal, slow-growing cancers (which are common in the elderly) are very risky. And the many women who are forced to live with the repercussions of false-positive mammograms have heightened levels of anxiety and other untoward psychological trauma.[23] Medicare's quality indicators do not advocate such screening over the age of seventy-five. But Medicare continues to pay for the test regardless of age, and has not used its guidelines to discourage screening mammograms in the oldest patients, which would seem more appropriate.

Screening for Everything

Bone density testing, something that is promoted by clinical guidelines and required by Medicare's quality measures for all women over age sixty-five, is a screening test that most of my patients feel is important. But those who get the test, some of them annually, have not considered how they would treat abnormal results, as many refuse to take the medicines that would be necessitated by a diagnosis of osteoporosis. In fact, they are correct to be skeptical of treatment, since bisphosphonates, the primary means of treating abnormal bone density tests, are of limited efficacy and have many adverse effects,[24] something we discussed in the prior chapter. In addition, no randomized studies have demonstrated long-term benefit from bone density testing.[25] In women with a normal bone density test, it would take fifteen years for 2 percent of them to develop a vertebral fracture,[26] making it questionable to even recommend subsequent testing in such patients. Thus, a well-regarded test that is believed to be a vital part of thorough medical screening, and that is both paid for and *encouraged* by Medicare through its clinical performance measures, does not necessarily lead to any meaningful enhancement of health in the vast majority of people who undergo it, but can expose women to potentially dangerous medicines. The test also labels many women with a diagnosis of osteoporosis, so now these women think they have a disease. In fact, by recently changing the definition of what is considered to be an abnormal bone density, more women now think they have osteoporosis, despite the fact that the new definitions of low bone density do not predispose people to additional clinically relevant fractures.[27]

Colonoscopies are also tests that are recommended for many patients but are controversial in their utility. My grandfather died from a colon prep, so I admit to being a bit skeptical. He was in his seventies, had serious heart disease, but still had a colonoscopy for routine screening that showed either a very large polyp or an early cancer, either of which required surgery to remove. So he went to the hospital feeling well, drank the gallon of GoLYTELY solution that night in preparation for the surgery, and was found dead on the floor the next morning. Likely that prep, which tears the body apart by pulling electrolytes from every cell imaginable, pushed his heart beyond his limit. An unnecessary test did him in. Many of my patients have had their bowels punctured by colon screening, being forced to have major surgery and then wear a bag to collect their stool. Some die. I have had other patients discover polyps that may become cancer, and they regard the test as lifesaving. But the reality is much different for our elderly,[28] where the risks of serious complications increase dramatically even as the benefits of screening diminish. In fact, it is felt that about a third of all cancer screening in the elderly is inappropriate.[29] These studies and others demonstrate that the number of lives saved from colon cancer detection with colonoscopy (approximately .25/1000 people screened in a year) is lower than the major complications, including perforation, that may result from screening (approximately 2.5/1000 people screened in a year). That is why so many organizations, including the US Preventive Services Task Force, do not endorse colon screening over age seventy-five, something echoed by Medicare's quality indicators. But many patients still believe scopes are necessary, despite their potential harm, and Medicare will gladly pay for the test, any complications that occur because of the test, and whatever treatments may be offered to ameliorate what diseases are uncovered. Again, Medicare could use its quality indicators to discourage such screening, but it does not.

A screening test that's become popular and widely talked about is CT scans for smokers and ex-smokers flowing from the results of a large randomized study, the National Lung Screening Trial (NLST). I have rarely met a smoker who does not think that they may get lung cancer; they often tell me that they would rather die of lung cancer than quit smoking. But now medical science has devised a means of preventing them from having to make that choice. A 2011 study showed that by performing annual high-definition CT scans on smokers and ex-smokers we can detect cancer early and save lives. The truth is much less spectacular when absolute risk reduction is looked at instead of the oft-published relative risk reduction,[30] but that did not stop the press from declaring the discovery a triumph of medical science, or Medicare from agreeing to pay for the test at enormous cost. In fact, despite a 20 percent relative risk reduction touted by the article results, the absolute risk reduction in lung cancer death was 3.3/1000 people screened over five years. Of people screened, almost a quarter had false-positive CT screens that were proven not to be cancer after further tests, some of which were invasive and potentially dangerous.[31] The US Preventive Services Task Force, which now recommends CT screening, cites a false-positive rate of almost 70 percent, and states that 9/1000 people who are screened are subjected to unnecessary biopsies or surgeries for benign lesions.[32] A subsequent look at the NLST data suggested that 18 percent of all cancers removed were indolent: if left alone, they would not have grown and thus would have caused no harm.[33]

CT screening, then, while showing a small reduction in lung cancer mortality, also confers substantial risk, especially in exposing large numbers of screened people to unnecessary procedures and treatments. It is also unclear if the results obtained in the ideal environment of NLST study centers can be generalized, or if the survival benefit will extend beyond five years, especially since smokers have a higher mortality rate from other causes. But CT screening is of dubious value for other reasons too. For one, the test gives patients the illusion that science is invincible and can cure even the most pesky problems. Smokers may come to expect the technological brilliance of our medical system will keep them from dying of lung cancer, and thus the quit rate may decline. Second, there are multiple risks with scanning. More than half of smokers over fifty years old have nodules on CT scans. Most nodules detected will never become cancers, yet to prove that, patients may undergo biopsies that can pop their lungs, cause infection, and even kill them. There is also no evidence prior to the recent study that following such nodules through serial CT scans is lifesaving or otherwise beneficial.[34] Also, there is a radiation risk associated with CT screening estimated to cause as many as 12/10,000 deaths in smokers screened.[35] Thus, because of an abnormal CT, some patients who do not have disease will be subjected to harm, even death, unnecessarily; many will be labeled with and treated for diseases that are not dangerous; and all are given the false promise that medical science can ameliorate even the most vexing health-care issues that plague us. Finally, generalized screening of smokers with CT scans will be very expensive and further tax Medicare while likely providing marginal, if any, absolute risk improvement once long-term data become available.

An editorial by Patrick Hahn in the *Baltimore Sun* states that the cost of "the illusion of cheating death" with lung cancer screening will be in the billions of dollars every year. This for perhaps a marginal extension of life, at best. As Professor Hahn poignantly says about patients who demand such testing: "On the one hand, too many people cannot be bothered to practice the behaviors that don't cost anyone else a penny, and which have proved to promote health and longevity: exercising, eating sensibly, and refraining from smoking and excess drinking. On the other hand, they demand endless, expensive medical interventions—not just regardless of cost, and not just regardless of how great a role their own foolishness has played in bringing on their disease, but regardless of whether said medical interventions are doing anyone any good."[36] To me, that sums it up perfectly.

What little evidence does support screening in the elderly is itself of questionable validity. Screening research tends to recruit better-educated people with fewer medical problems, and these studies are subject to multiple biases.[37] One of my colleagues, Erik Rifkin, the author of *The Illusion of Certainty*, has written a book that explores multiple medical interventions in absolute terms. In *Interpreting Health Benefits and Risks* he utilizes a 1,000-seat theater (benefit/risk characterization theater, or BRCT) to demonstrate how many people benefit and are harmed by over twenty medical tests, procedures, and treatments. For instance, the benefit of smokers who quit smoking essentially fills every seat of the theater (they all benefit), while doing a colonoscopy in an asymptomatic person will help two people in the theater, and hurt two other people in the theater. But when I show some of my patients the very dramatic theater presentation, they look at the two seats of people who avert colon cancer through screening and say, "One of those guys could be me. That's why I want the test." I point to the 998 seats of people who do not benefit from a colonoscopy, and the two seats of people who will get serious complications from the colonoscopy, some needing lifelong bags to empty their stool due to colon puncture, others dying from the procedure or prep. Still, many patients would rather take that chance. Medicare pays for the test. The doctor recommended it. Their kids insist on it. They don't want to die of colon cancer. And somehow this test, like so many others, will enable them to cheat death. It is a common human flaw to believe such magical thinking. And as long as Medicare is paying, then what the hell.

X-rays and Other Scans

In our technologically advanced society doctors can employ the power of radiation and magnets (X-rays, CT scans, MRIs, etc.) to look into the body and find trouble. Then, as with numbers that are outside the "normal" range, we can make everything better again with enough effort, probing, and slicing. Very few see the danger of digging too deep and then repairing what is wrong. Says one doctor who studies health-care delivery: "If a procedure or surgery helps you, you proclaim how lucky you are to live in such a medically advantaged country. If it doesn't work or you get hurt, you think your disease is just too much for modern medicine. If you die, your survivors blame the disease, not the procedure."[38]

Mr. L. came to me with back pain. He seemed to have strained his lumbar spine at the gym. He was healthy and vibrant, and we agreed to treat him with some physical therapy and medicines. But the back did not improve, so we ordered a simple back X-ray. Well, the bones were normal, and the back improved, but the X-ray showed some calcium in the abdomen that was in the area of his aorta, and they suggested we order an ultrasound. So we did. And in fact he had a large aneurysm in his aorta. I sent him to a specialist, who suggested that while the aneurysm (called an AAA, or abdominal aortic aneurysm) had not caused the back pain (which it sometimes can), it was just too big to leave alone. So Mr. L. went for surgery, and Mr. L. died in surgery. A simple back X-ray that should never have been ordered opened Pandora's box. We screen for AAAs, especially in smokers, and we often find them incidentally, but there is minimal evidence that such a proactive approach reduces mortality.[39] As with Mr. L., it is often best to leave well enough alone. That is not to say that all tests lead us down a dangerous road, as in the case of Mr. L. But we should be cautious when we test, because false-positive findings and the discovery of diseases that are best left alone can lead to adverse outcomes if pursued. In many of our tests, especially as patients become older, the majority of "positive" results are not helpful, or are frankly harmful.

It is estimated that two-thirds of MRIs ordered contribute nothing to patient care. In fact, like with Mr. L., we uncover "problems" for which we are not searching, leading to more tests, procedures, and potential harm. One study showed that 87 percent of whole-body scans found abnormalities, 40 percent required more testing, and less than 1 percent revealed any clinically relevant information after all the testing was complete.[40] In people without any symptoms, random X-rays revealed gallstones in 10 percent of people tested, old strokes in 10 percent, cartilage damage to the knees in 40 percent, and bulging back disks in 50 percent.[41] Knee imaging poorly predicts clinically relevant illness, especially in the elderly, and contributes virtually nothing to help improve outcome or symptoms in patients with knee pain.[42] In addition, despite their limited utility, some studies suggest that the radiation exposure inflicted by such tests as CT scans can actually directly harm patients; the National Cancer Institute estimated that in a single year CT radiation caused 29,000 excess cases of cancer and 14,500 excess deaths.[43] And yet these tests are commonly requested and ordered; they are considered thorough care for many Americans. And Medicare pays for them; I have never seen a request for a scan denied in my twenty years of practice.

Many illnesses, especially cancers, have become more prevalent in our society because imaging and testing have revealed tumors that previously would have gone undetected. But although we have diagnosed more cancer, we have not seen improvement in survival rates. For instance, the diagnosis of kidney cancer has increased dramatically from 1975 to the present, but there has been no change in kidney cancer deaths. Some of these increased numbers of kidney cancer were found incidentally on CT scans done for other reasons, and they may not have caused harm. Because so many kidney tumors are identified, many people have had to endure unnecessary, potentially dangerous procedures and surgeries to remove tumors that may have been harmless if left alone.[44] In fact, autopsy studies demonstrate that in 25–40 percent of cases, patients die from causes that differ from their diagnosis,[45] a diagnosis often made as the result of a radiologic test that should not have been ordered.

When to Test: The Case of Back Pain

The perception that MRIs will help a person with back pain is common among my patients, but the data for such a presumption is at best specious.[46] For an excellent analysis of this, I suggest reading Richard Deyo's book *Watch Your Back,* which explores the illusion that testing and treating people with back pain improves outcome. Many of my patients with back pain ask for back MRIs, despite my advice otherwise. There are certainly times when an MRI makes sense: when pain persists despite every effort to curb it, when neurologic damage is evident, and when the test may reveal some finding that is pragmatically treatable. But we should get the MRI only if we are looking for something that can be fixed, and for which the patient is willing to undergo available treatment. Only one in 2,500 MRIs provides information that is not uncovered by the patient's history, and less than 1 percent of all scans show cancer, typically in people with either a past history of cancer or who have other symptoms or signs of cancer.[47] Virtually none of these cancers are curable, even if discovered by testing. Overall, 75 percent of people with lower back pain make a full recovery within three months without treatment, and there is no change in this number if they have received an MRI.[48] And several studies have demonstrated that there is no improvement in outcome or psychological wellbeing in people who receive an MRI compared to those who do not. In fact, just the opposite may be true. MRIs done within the first month of symptoms can lead to worse outcomes and unnecessary surgery.[49] But why not test and find the precise cause of the pain? After all, it is better to obtain more information and find out what is going on rather than guess. That is thorough medicine.

In fact, when MRIs are done on populations of people with back pain and those without back pain, both groups are found to have similar disk problems in their back regardless of whether they have pain. Ninety percent of *asymptomatic* people over the age of sixty have spinal abnormalities on MRI, including spinal stenosis, bulging disks, and even herniated disks.[50] This is a tremendously high false-positive rate. Of course, the patients with back pain claim that the bulging disk uncovered by the MRI is causing their pain, when in fact it may have been there quietly for years and has nothing to do with why they are hurting. If we find a slipped disk, and we have already exhausted common treatments such as physical therapy and medicine, then potentially the patient can have cortisone injections or even surgery. But will that treatment work, and will the patients want that treatment? If the answers are no, then there is no purpose for getting the MRI. Many studies have demonstrated the futility of invasively treating most back pain.[51] One study suggested that 10 percent more people with back pain did better long term *without* cortisone injections in the back compared to those who had injections.[52] Thus treatment that is performed explicitly as a result of an MRI and which itself carries some risk, as we learned from the fungal-infected injections that killed people recently, has dubious value and can cause harm, especially since the vast majority of people improve without any testing or treatment.

In the world of medical common sense, certain means exist to evaluate the utility of a test. First of all the test should be performed to look for a specific condition, not just to look around and see what is brewing. When we look around we often uncover conditions not related to the patient's complaint, and that sends us down a very precarious road. Second, the patient should have a high pretest probability of having that condition—in other words, a clinical state that makes the condition very likely. When the pretest probability is low, then the likelihood is that whatever the test reveals may not be the cause of the patient's problem or could be false positives. In addition, the test needs to add information that a medical history or physical exam will not reveal. Third, the condition for which we are testing will be harmful if left alone and will worsen without intervention. Fourth, an intervention exists to fix the problem, the patients would want to pursue that intervention, and the intervention is less dangerous than the condition itself if left alone.

Unfortunately, common sense is often absent from both our current dogma of what constitutes thorough medical care and how Medicare finances that care. It is far easier for us as doctors to just order a test than to engage in a complicated conversation with our patients about the ramifications of testing. Medicare will reimburse doctors well for testing, but it does not pay adequately for that type of discussion.

Cardiac Testing

Cardiac testing is especially illustrative of how Americans perceive tests and procedures as being beneficial despite evidence to the contrary. Many of my patients expect an EKG as part of their annual exam, and many more see cardiologists where they receive regular cardiac testing—EKGs, echocardiograms, stress tests, Holter monitors—as part of routine surveillance. Such testing seems both innocuous and thorough, and most of my patients are glad to be so well cared for by their doctors. However, while 700,000 Medicare patients reported receiving annual treadmill stress tests in 2008 (and the numbers continue to climb), such tests poorly predict both who has serious disease and who has no disease.[53] In fact, while 1.9/1000 may have disease detected by stress testing that, if treated, will improve their outcome, 6.5 people out of one thousand with low-risk nuclear stress tests will have cardiac death or heart attack in a year despite being told their tests are normal, and two in one thousand people tested will actually suffer an excessive risk of death, heart attack, and stroke (from unnecessary procedures done based on the very high rate of false positive tests) simply from getting a stress test they did not need. There may even be an increased risk of cancer due to radiation exposure.[54] The numbers are not very different in CT angiograms, which are the newest version of testing people for cardiac disease. Thus, such testing often misses those with real disease, and also causes unnecessary death and disability in people who should never have received the test in the first place.

Mr. S., who is in his seventies, is not a big fan of tests, but he was pushed to have one out of necessity. Not that he was feeling poorly; he was not. He was a pilot who continued to relish trips into the clouds, and he paid for his hobby by teaching flying lessons at the local airport. He was excellent at what he did, and it gave his life a meaning and purpose that allowed him to thrive. But one day a new FAA doctor looked at his EKG for his annual flight exam and thought it seemed abnormal. In fact, it had always been abnormal, and Mr. S. pulled out a very old EKG to demonstrate that fact. But the doctor insisted on more testing, and he ordered a flurry of tests from a cardiologist, including a thallium stress test, all of which Medicare paid for. Understand, Mr. S. has no heart symptoms and few risk factors, and the test was done only because of an EKG that had not changed in decades. But when the thallium test was read as being abnormal, now he was told he had a serious illness.

It was not markedly abnormal, and even the cardiologist accepted that it may be a normal variant. So he ordered a CT angiogram, which also demonstrated equivocal results. Then he ordered a cardiac catheterization (itself a potentially dangerous procedure), which showed a blockage of one artery, though not necessarily the artery suspected to be blocked based on the prior tests. Still, the cardiologist recommended surgery to fix the artery, since the narrowing was not amenable to the placement of a stent. Mr. S., knowing that only the surgery would get him in the air again, reluctantly complied.

The surgery proved complicated. Mr. S. has a decades-long platelet problem, meaning that his blood does not clot well. So he bled excessively. Then his prostate expanded and he could not urinate. He needed a urinary catheter placed, and had to go home with it and with nurses to take care of it. When they attempted to remove the catheter, his prostate continued to block his urine flow. This went on for months, until finally he needed another surgery to open the prostate. Over the course of this his stress level escalated, and he became progressively more debilitated. Months passed before he could function well again. And when they checked his heart tests again, there had been no change. Nothing improved. They still denied him his license. The surgery likely did nothing to prevent a heart attack or to extend his life. In fact, it only induced pain and misery, increased his stress and disability, and potentially caused him great harm. A door was yanked open that should have been kept closed. And Mr. S. was the victim of the abuse of thorough.

What is the evidence that cardiac testing—stress tests, echocardiograms, catheterizations—helps reveal problems whose resolution leads to saved lives? When elderly patients are having chest pains or shortness of breath, should they see cardiologists, get procedures, have blocked vessels fixed by stents or surgery? So many of my patients get stress tests on a regular basis, sometimes even every year. Some of them have symptoms, some had symptoms or heart problems in the past, some just want to make sure everything is OK. There are clearly medicines that help prevent heart attacks in patients with certain conditions, some of which may be defined through cardiac testing, so there is a rationale for targeted testing of specific people. We do know that in certain types of heart disease, invasive procedures such as bypass and stenting can be lifesaving.

But the basis for conducting many heart tests may rest on faulty grounds, as we have discussed.[55] Even if one argues that a stress test or echocardiogram can reveal a problem that will lead to beneficial treatment, one still has to follow the rules of what constitutes a good reason for testing, as I outlined above. And that certainly does not justify the frequency of cardiac testing that is being inflicted on many of my older patients. In the elderly, heart disease is omnipresent, but that does not mean it is lethal or even damaging, or that repairing the problem will improve clinical outcome, or even that the procedures used to fix problems are not more dangerous than the problems themselves. Many people have blockages in their arteries, but that does not necessarily mean that they are at risk for cardiac death. Some people, probably like Mr. S., develop collateral circulation around the blockages, and a majority of people who have serious cardiac events such as sudden death and heart attacks have relatively minor blockages not detected by stress testing.[56] And the vast majority of heart attacks occur in blood vessels that do not have blockages; finding a blockage and fixing it does not protect most people from getting a heart attack. In fact, calculating a calcium score based on an inexpensive CT scan (about $70) better · predicts who is at low and high risk of heart attack regardless of there being any blockages to fix.[57] But we can find heart disease if we look, even if that heart disease is not clinically relevant and even if the treatment of that disease may cause more harm than good. And we are certainly looking very hard!

Many of my patients have had heart attacks at some time in their lives, from fairly significant events, to minor blockages, to silent myocardial infarctions (MIs). Many of my patients recount tales of getting to the hospital just in time, being saved by the doctors there, and lauding the thorough care that kept them alive then and for time immemorial. But is aggressive testing and treatment after a heart attack as beneficial as my patients surmise? The answer may well be no.[58] After an MI in the United States, doctors perform an increased number of invasive tests and vessel-opening procedures (catheters, stents, bypass surgeries) than do doctors of similar patients in Canada, but the one year mortality rate is equal in both countries.[59] The regional variations in this country are also striking. Medicare patients in Texas are 50 percent more likely than those in New York to be catheterized within ninety days of an MI with an added cost of $10,000 per patient. However, despite such thorough care, outcomes are worse in Texas than in New York, with increased death and increased injury.[60] Even in people who have not had heart attacks, doctors in the United States perform excessive numbers of catheterizations, stents, and bypass surgeries for symptoms and conditions for which there is not always medical justification. It is estimated that of the 1.2 million elective cardiac procedures, 160,000 or more are not appropriate.[61]

Opening Blocked Arteries: Stents and Bypass

If we find a blocked artery, should we fix it in the elderly? Does opening an artery extend one's life, or, like with Mr. S., is it a potentially unnecessary procedure with serious complications that does not extend life or reduce symptoms? So many of my patients are walking around with bypassed arteries and multiple stents. They perceive that they would be dead without those procedures. Much of what we know through the literature would dispute that assumption. In fact, in most situations, inexpensive medicines and lifestyle changes are as or more effective than aggressive and expensive cardiac procedures such as stents and bypass surgery.[62] Some would argue that stents and bypass cause more harm than good, and that looking for and fixing blockages is bad medicine, especially for the elderly. We know too that finding blocked heart valves or leaking valves will not necessarily lead to a treatment that will confer any benefit unless that patient has such severe symptoms that no other option exists.[63]

It seems logical that if a doctor orders a stress test and, after additional testing such as catheterization, discovers a blocked artery that leads to the heart, then opening that artery will be beneficial, especially if it can be accomplished just by inserting a metal stent. After all, isn't an open artery better than a closed one, and isn't it sensible to search for closed arteries and then perform a simple procedure to open them? Stenting is illustrative of a medical logic that convinces so many patients to pursue tests and treatments that seem reasonable and life saving but in fact are often just the opposite. Unfortunately, far more than people realize, medical truth often is counterintuitive. In fact, unless heart blockages are in a few very specific arteries in the heart, stents not only do not save people's lives but actually they can cause harm. Many people bypass their own blocked arteries, so stenting them accomplishes nothing other than exposing them to an unnecessary procedure and dangerous medicines. Many of those who have heart attacks do so even after the stent is placed, in an artery that was not even identified as being blocked at the time of the stress test. The vast majority of people with heart disease reduce their chance of getting a heart attack more by taking a few inexpensive medicines than by putting in a stent since, as we have stated already, most (over 80 percent) of heart attacks occur in blood vessels that are not blocked and thus cannot be fixed with a stent. And the vast majority of people with blocked arteries will not get a heart attack and thus do not need a stent. Looking and finding and opening heart arteries in people without symptoms seems amazing and life saving but, as studies cited above show, all too often simply expose patient to unnecessary risk. And yet Medicare dollars continue to flow to the expansive and financially bloated stenting industry that enriches doctors and hospitals and device makers but rarely ever helps the patients who believe their lives were saved. Meanwhile, both Medicare and the grateful patients with stents neglect the most effective and inexpensive paths to heart health—nutrition, exercise, stress reduction, and good primary care. This is a paradox that is emblematic of the type of erroneous thinking that pushes Medicare down a very dangerous precipitance, both for its financial survivability and for the patients it is trying to serve.

Even when people sail through elective cardiac procedures, and even though they are typically convinced that they would have died without such timely intervention, testing and treatment is not without risk. There is good evidence that people who undergo open heart surgery suffer mental decline.[64] People can bleed, develop cardiac complications, have sudden heart attacks and strokes, acquire infections, and sustain organ damage from cardiac tests and procedures. Some never regain their prior level of function, especially the old and frail. All patients who undergo cardiac procedures now are labeled as cardiac patients, and this creates a psychological strain that impacts them for the rest of their lives. Some see themselves as being sick, and thus subject themselves to even more tests and procedures, a venture financed by Medicare.

Mr. B. was a good looking, pleasant man with dementia in our retirement community, who lived from smile to smile and joke to joke. His debonair southern accent (his family hailed from New Orleans, where they owned a large part of that city from well before the Civil War) wooed women, young and old, thus provoking ire in his wife. He often wandered to the medical center to spend time with us.

Mr. B.'s most pressing medical problem was shortness of breath from a leaky heart valve. He saw a ton of specialists, had an abundance of tests performed regularly, and was on a drawerful of medicines (which he took when he felt like it), but nothing fully alleviated his symptoms. He never complained about his breathing; other people were more concerned about it than he was. He took his time getting from one place to another with frequent rests and, as he explained, he had ample time, so that was no problem. At the retirement community in which he lived he could do anything he wanted, including frequently visiting us, panting a bit, but always with a smile and a joke. When I asked him if he was OK, he would say, "Sure, I can still play my cornet; when I can't do that, I know I am in trouble."

He always talked about his cornet and the bands he had played with in New Orleans. We never knew if he really still played it or whether it was an echo from his past. Then one day he marched down to the medical center with a black box, pulled out his gold cornet, and belted out some tunes, with a pitch as smooth and suave as Mr. B. himself. Everyone gathered around to listen to his show, in which he sprinkled several jokes and stories. Mr. B. loved an audience, and he soaked up the attention. On many days after that, he would show up with his cornet.

Although I saw Mr. B. fairly often, typically at the behest of his wife, or as an excuse for him to come down and mingle with the ladies, he never complained. Never. He did not have an ache or pain, never a sad thought, never a flicker of distress. But his wife worried, especially about his breathing. She brought him from specialist to specialist. They pushed her to have him repair his leaky heart valve, something Mr. B. bucked until finally the pressure to be aggressive became overwhelming to him. So he agreed to the procedure, probably just to shut everyone up.

I remember the day before his surgery. Mr. B. walked down to see us with his toothy grin, his smooth one-liners, and his cornet. He played a few tunes for us, never gasping for air, and hung around for a while before meeting his wife at dinner, which started at about 4:00 p.m. That was the last I saw him. Several days later we learned that Mr. B. had died in the hospital. The lifesaving surgery had triggered a cascade of other problems from which he could not recover.

Mr. M. was a short-statured man who liked to meander down to our medical center to chat with the receptionists or whoever else was willing to talk. Like Mr. B., he would often toss them a joke or a funny story in his gruff voice. He had been a working man all his life, not particularly well educated or well spoken, but always upbeat and outgoing. His wife, also a fount of pleasantness, was more reserved, playing the straight man to his comedic routine.

For any number of reasons—small strokes, cerebral atrophy, arthritis, neuropathy, blocked blood vessels in his heart—Mr. M. began to lose his balance and become more short of breath. He fell often, and became unable to traverse long distances, even with a walker. Frequently his wife pushed him to the medical center or to dinner in a wheelchair, which not only felt demeaning to Mr. M., but threatened his spontaneity and independence. I did the requisite CT scan of his brain and some labs. We ordered physical therapy, played with his medicines, tried some tricks, but his balance continued to decline and his breathing worsened. And so, as I often do in such circumstances, I shrugged my shoulders.

"Hey doc, should I see a neurologist or do something else or is this it?" Mr. M. asked me.

I told him the truth. Fifteen years of experience with neurologists taught me a harsh reality: they were excellent at labeling diseases, but terrible at treating them.

"What about my breathing? Could it be my heart, doc? Everyone tells me I should get my heart looked at."

I told him that it was possible. It was also possible that his leg weakness caused him to be unable to exercise, which led him to be out of shape. We could send him to a heart doctor, do some tests, possibly put him on some medicines, but those would have side effects. He may also be sent down a road littered with invasive procedures.

"Then I don't got time for that. You tell me. What do we do?"

Mr. M. eschewed testing and treatments; he was a hands-off kind of guy. Had it not been for the fact that Mr. M. frequently mocked people who rode around the halls recklessly in their electric wheelchairs, then maybe I would have suggested such a chair as a possible solution. I did not. But Mrs. M. did. They bickered about it for several of our subsequent visits, between which Mr. M., determined as ever, tried to walk and nearly broke his hip. Finally, with goading from both of us, he relented. Of course, that was the easy part. I then had to tackle pages upon pages of papers to convince Medicare that an electric wheelchair was justified. That is no simple task. Today it would even be less feasible.

For a while we did not see much of Mr. M. But then one day he emerged in the medical center on his shiny red, brand-new Hoveround wheelchair with which Medicare, after weeks of struggle, had graciously provided him. He mocked himself, pretending to be lame, talking like an old man. And then he showed off his moves, rapid turns, and high-speed sprints down the medical center halls. Soon after that he purchased an electric message display—a smaller version of the screen over Times Square—and welded it to the front of his chair. He became a fixture all over the retirement community. He broadcast holidays, birthdays, events, and even jokes on his chair's display. On various holidays he dressed himself up as Santa, or a leprechaun, or in colonial garb, and he decorated his chair too.

As the years passed, Mrs. M. died suddenly of cancer, and Mr. M.'s health deteriorated. He still pulled himself into that chair every day, always with some purpose like delivering a message or new joke, and he made the rounds, honking his horn to announce his arrival with a smile on his face. The chair allowed him to stay in his apartment and avoid a move to an assisted-living facility or nursing home. Mr. M. died peacefully in his sleep one night. He was in his nineties, and just as happy as the first day I met him.

Medicare paid $5,000 for Mr. M.'s wheelchair after a lot of paperwork and arm twisting. That wheelchair saved Medicare a ton of cash; one trip to the emergency room for a fall or for shortness of breath often costs much more than that, and a hip fracture or cardiac procedure costs tens of thousands of dollars more. But more important, that wheelchair enhanced his life immeasurably and allowed him to preserve his humor and dignity to the end. Had Mr. M. raced from test to test and specialist to specialist, had he been dragged to the emergency room for falls, had he broken his hip and required weeks of inpatient rehabilitation, had he had cardiac tests and stents placed (because certainly if we looked we would have found heart disease that could be treated), Medicare would have paid without batting an eye. Instead Medicare paid for his inexpensive and life-sustaining chair reluctantly and after great effort. Medicare paid Mr. B.'s tab, however, without any question or hassle, at a likely cost of tens of thousands of dollars and at the cost of his life.

So often I watch as patients and families make the difficult choices that fell on Mr. B. and Mr. M. And so often they leap on the path of thorough care. They try to fix persistent problems, some of which are found by testing and cause no or minimal symptoms, by utilizing the most draconian and invasive methods available. They try to eradicate illness, such as cancers and heart disease, that if left alone are almost always less toxic than the cures. For many patients, families, and doctors the curative, aggressive approach often seems like the right path at first, but rarely does it lead to good outcomes. People justify their decisions by thinking that they have no choice, and indeed the price is often cheaper to the patient to take the most aggressive approach (even if it does cost society a fortune). Medicare makes it easier to be more aggressive; it will not finance help at home and may pay for medical equipment that can improve quality of life, but only after a time-consuming paperwork battle. Meanwhile, Medicare readily pays for tests and procedures, typically with little effort by the patient's doctor. But like with Mr. M., sometimes the least invasive fix is most beneficial. If only Medicare agreed!

Dialysis

Kidney disease is another illness that is fairly common in the elderly and will be detected if we look hard enough. Many of my older patients have some degree of kidney impairment, and knowing that it will not impact their lives, I typically ignore it. But many doctors are far more thorough in testing and treating patients with any degree of renal decline. When patients get pushed onto the train of aggressive kidney surveillance, often at the behest of a kidney doctor (nephrologist) whom they choose to see, they are often barraged by tests, given handfuls of medicines of questionable benefit, and told that dialysis is in their futures. Most of my patients put in this category now have to live with an unnecessary stress that their kidneys can fail at any time. When the kidneys do fail, they are told that they will have to receive dialysis.

Dialysis is not easy, and it is life altering. For three days a week patients go to a dialysis center, have a large needle inserted in a surgically created fistula in their arm, and lie there for many hours as their blood is circulated through an artificial kidney. Very often their blood pressure drops very low, their body chemicals flurry into disarray, and they feel miserable for that day and typically the next. Many of my patients are whisked from the dialysis center to the hospital due to emergencies that dialysis inflicts on their fragile bodies. Some acquire infections or catastrophic difficulties with their shunts. Suffice it to say that while dialysis may be lifesaving for some, it is life destroying for many,[65] and I truly am amazed at how quickly some of my patients are hurried into dialysis with little medical justification for so draconian an approach. Again, as with cardiac patients, many of these patients are thankful for their lives being saved by the miracle of dialysis, whether true or not, and despite the marked decline in life quality many of them must endure, while others truly need dialysis for symptom relief or to stay alive. Still, I have seen nursing-home residents with dementia and weak elderly patients forced to travel to a dialysis center three days a week, wiped out and exhausted, more confused, more ill than before. There seems to be no limit as to who is offered this expensive and debilitating, but very profitable, procedure. And many of them likely would have lived healthy, vibrant lives had they simply been left alone. We have no data to indicate otherwise, and my experience has shown this to be the case.

Medicare pays well for dialysis. In fact, doctors who place their patients on dialysis are likely to be financially rewarded. There are few hard criteria that Medicare requires before dialysis is instigated, and Medicare more readily pays for that procedure than for the much lower cost of helping a kidney-failure patient stay off dialysis machines.

This year I took care of a wonderful man in his eighties who had moved to a local assisted-living facility after starting dialysis. He left friends, including a girlfriend, and a life he truly enjoyed to be closer to his daughter and to a dialysis center. He was emotionally beaten and physically torn apart by the dialysis. I tried to ascertain why he needed dialysis, and why it had to be given three days a week, since that wiped him out almost the entire week. For some reason many kidney doctors insist that anyone who starts dialysis get treatment three days a week, no matter how severe their kidney dysfunction is. I have also found that some people who start dialysis, especially older people, are doing just fine with their poorly functioning kidneys, and it is only excessive testing, excessive medicine use, and specialist involvement that pushes them across the rocky precipice to accept a treatment that is both potentially dangerous and debilitating while often being of questionable clinical efficacy. Mr. B. seemed to fit into that category. He still made urine. His labs were not terrible. He had no fluid overload. Still, his doctors insisted that he needed dialysis and they convinced him and his family that without dialysis his life was in peril. Just a few weeks ago Mr. B. developed problems with his dialysis shunt, the surgically created blood vessel into which a dialysis needle is placed during treatments. It shut off and became infected, and he needed another catheter placed into his chest to continue his dialysis treatment. He started getting weaker and more depressed. Then, as I learned the other day, he went in for a minor surgery to fix the shunt, and he died.

In reality, Mr. B. was dying before the procedure killed him; his life had been torn apart by his "need" for dialysis. But did he really need it? From my review of his record, he did not. He was put on dialysis because his numbers had become worse, even as he continued to live a happy and vibrant life. If his clinical situation worsened, something that I have found to be relatively uncommon in the very oldest of our patients, he may have chosen to endure dialysis at that juncture. Or perhaps he would have preferred a palliative approach with home health aides and fluid management, and he could have remained at home with his friends and his life left intact. Although that less thorough approach is inexpensive compared to dialysis, Medicare is not willing to help pay for it. It is more than willing to pay the total bill for dialysis and for all of Mr. B.'s surgeries, including the one that ultimately killed him. That bill is exorbitant, financially and personally. The cost was the man's happiness, health, and ultimately his life.

Procedures of All Forms

Like with heart disease and kidney disease, many elderly people have medical problems that are revealed by testing and can be potentially fixed with procedures. Most elderly people urinate too much. Some men have enlarged prostates, some men and woman have spastic bladders. High-tech testing can measure urinary flow and even prostate size. Bladder scopes can examine the inner lining of the bladder, the flow, and the precise squeeze pressures of the various components of the bladder. Patients then can be treated with various surgeries for either the prostate or bladder. Recently a patient of mine received Botox injections in her bladder to help spasm. As a result she had complete loss of urinary function for three months, requiring a permanent catheter. Other patients have bladder-lifting surgery, which typically affords them a few months of relief before it collapses again at the cost of exposing their bodies to anesthesia and a surgeon's knife.[66] Typically urinary problems can be diagnosed by doctors like me without any testing, and they can be managed with behavior therapy, minor life adjustments, and the use of pads to soak up leaking urine, and often some generic medicine. When conservative treatment fails, and if the symptoms are sufficiently severe, then we may consider tests and treatments. Medicare pays for the aggressive care without blinking an eye. To get it to pay for diapers is a far more difficult venture!

From painful neuropathy in the feet, to acid reflux and swallowing problems, to arthritis and constipation, we have expensive tests to dig into every issue that is common among the elderly. The tests can help define the problems, label patients with specific diagnoses that they can carry with them in their pockets, and afford these patients confidence that they have been thoroughly worked up for their maladies. Typically the testing doctor will offer patients various treatments, some more invasive than others, and most only questionably effective. Many elderly people in our society live with the assumption that if a disease can be defined, then it can be ameliorated. But such thinking is financially costly and medically risky. Prunes help constipation, and exercise certainly helps arthritis; we do not need sophisticated tests and scientific explanations to figure that out. Unfortunately, in our test-crazed society, common sense and an acceptance of aging quickly evaporate when more technologically sophisticated methods are so readily available for free.

There are of course many examples where testing and treatment make sense and produce favorable results. I have seen people undergo bypass surgery because of persistent pain and shortness of breath that cannot be relieved with medication and behavior changes, and the result is an improvement in their quality of life. One patient who did everything to avoid cardiac surgery, including taking far too many medicines and driving an electric cart, simply had a disease far too severe for him to flourish, preventing him from sleeping at night, going to the bathroom, and visiting his wife at a nursing home. When finally he made the decision to have surgery, he did so because he preferred death over his current condition. The surgery allowed him to function again, and although he lived only another year before he died, he told me that it was the best year he ever had. The price tag for that surgery was high, and it did not buy him extra time to live, but it did accomplish something positive.

Similarly, I have had patients who get dizzy and pass out with high frequency, and after testing they are often found to need pacemakers. Those pacemakers can essentially cure them. One of my patients walked around with a heart rate in the 40s and felt tired. For years he fought getting a pacemaker, but when he finally ended up in the hospital due to passing out, and he agreed to have the pacemaker placed, he woke up with more energy than he had had since he was a kid. Another patient fainted incessantly, and thousands of dollars of testing and even a few hospital visits did not define what caused her to do so. Finally, after she passed out while driving and hit a tree, breaking several bones, a monitor in the emergency room happened to show that her heart periodically stopped for several seconds. She had a pacemaker placed, and never passed out again.

Other patients become dysfunctional from arthritis, and despite multiple conservative treatments are unable to live with any quality. For many, joint replacements give them the ability to live again. Some patients need procedures to dilate their esophagus periodically to help them swallow, and only with testing and treatment can that be achieved. Many patients develop a condition where they stop breathing at night (sleep apnea), the results of which are fatigue and heart strain. Testing and treatment (wearing a difficult-to-use mask at night called a CPAP) can help dramatically. Sleep apnea is a good example of how testing and treatment can help, but also how it is bereft of nuance. Often patients can cure their sleep apnea by losing weight, and no test can help with that. Certain behavior therapies can help too. And very often, despite all the testing they have to endure, my patients refuse treatment, because the treatment itself can be very uncomfortable. And that brings us to where we started. We have to accept that certain maladies are common with age. Many of them can be mitigated and improved by accommodating them and carrying out simple behavioral changes. When they become too much of a burden, and when testing is done for a specific reason that may lead to a treatment the patient is willing to accept, and which is medically beneficial and safe, then that testing makes sense. But tests should not be done simply to be thorough. The pursuit of thorough is a prevalent, dangerous, and expensive idea that has no place in our geriatric medical dogma, even if Medicare is willing to pay.

Fishing: The Case of Dementia

Sometimes with age the body declines not only organ by organ, but also more globally. My oldest patients are more tired and more confused, they lose weight, they have less desire to interact and get out of their chairs, and they have a litany of complaints for which a cause cannot be ascertained. Often those problems emanate from their medical ailments or their medicines; people with poorly functioning hearts, for example, can experience fatigue and confusion from both the heart and the drugs used to treat the heart. Also quite frequently those problems are a manifestation of depression, which itself can be very difficult to treat although always worth a try. But many patients and families demand a more precise and thorough investigation into the physical and mental decline that occurs so frequently in the aged. Somehow, they reason, these symptoms are treatable, and something is underlying them. They want more answers.

"I want Dad to have a whole-body CT scan to figure out what is going on."

That statement, which is common in many renditions, is a request for us to go fishing. Let's throw our hook into the bay and see what we can snag. Then let's fix whatever we snag, and see if that resolves the problem. If Dad does not improve, we will keep throwing in our hooks, maybe even moving to different bodies of water, finding different captains to help us, never backing down until Dad gets better, like he was in the past. There is a solution if we are persistent and thorough enough.

Of course, disease-specific testing is itself problematic and must be done with care and common sense, but fishing is a geriatric nightmare. It seems to be most common among my most frail patients with the greatest degrees of dementia, typically those whose families have taken over their care, and it causes my patients stress and anguish rather than leading to any meaningful improvement.

Dementia is a prime example of how fishing is used to snag an imaginary resolution to a horrible ailment. When people become confused they may have simple memory loss common in aging, or they may have a progressive form of memory loss called dementia. Medical scientists have defined various forms of dementia, from Alzheimer's disease, to multi-infarct dementia (multiple tiny strokes), to Lewy body dementia (dementia with Parkinson's features), to frontal lobe dementia (striking mostly the front part of the brain and causing more behavior issues). As a geriatric doctor I find these categorizations to be unhelpful. First of all, there is no way to differentiate one from another based on hard evidence. Second, I have very few patients who fit into only one category, making me believe that dementia is more of a spectrum of disease that is most impacted by where it hits the brain the hardest. And third, whatever minimal treatments exist for these conditions are virtually the same regardless of how dementia is labeled.

Still, some patients and families seeking to better understand the cause and nature of the disease, to better be able to grapple with its progression and be better able to treat it, want concrete and scientific answers. Some of my patients' families run Mom to neurologists, often seek "experts" in academic medical centers, put Mom through a battery of tests, and then come to me and announce that Mom does not have dementia like I had told them, but rather she has Pick's disease (a form of dementia). I then ask how it is being treated. They proclaim that the experts are putting Mom on medicines that will help slow the disease, and that they intend to monitor Mom closely. Of course I have to just nod and smile, since I know there is no meaningful way to monitor Mom, that the medicines she is being put on are identical to ones that had previously been ineffective, and that more likely than not the medicines will not impact the disease meaningfully, as I have discussed in the prior chapter.

Just yesterday I was listening to a new NPR show when the host announced that in the next segment we would learn why if you or your loved one has been diagnosed with Alzheimer's disease you may want to get a second opinion. The host then interviewed an academic neurosurgeon who quite bluntly stated that 5 to 10 percent of alleged cases of dementia are misdiagnosed and are actually cases of NPH (normal pressure hydrocephalus), a condition of fluid buildup in the brain that is treated with a surgical procedure carried out by specialists such as the doctor being interviewed. The doctor explained that with treatment his patients shed their dementia and weakness and became normal again, sometimes instantly.[67]

In my twenty-year experience, I am aware of approximately five patients diagnosed with NPH among the thousands of dementia patients I have cared for. Talking to other geriatric doctors, I find we all have similar experiences. In fact, thorough testing, such as that performed by dementia specialists, will uncover a reversible problem in three out of one thousand people with dementia.[68] Much if not all of that testing has already been ordered by primary-care doctors like me. We typically perform scans to look for NPH, and we order lab tests to find other possibly reversible forms of dementia. Then, when those tests reveal nothing of substance, we have to confront the realities of dementia. Stories like this on NPR only send patients and their families on a quest for the impossible, one that typically ends in disappointment, if it ends at all. As we try to help our patients and families cope with dementia, the press, friends, and a few overly sanguine doctors tell them that they need to be more thorough. Just find another doctor and miracles will occur!

But in fact when testing will not accomplish something meaningful, and when no reasonable treatment exists as a result of that testing, I believe that being "thorough" leads us down a dangerous road. Families and patients are flooded with false hope. Patients are stressed by the process, something I have seen over and over in my practice, and that stress only exacerbates their dementia and detracts from their quality of life. Fishing for answers is not a very useful means of spending taxpayer funds, although many think it defines thorough, and although it is consistently paid for.

Excessive testing is rewarded in many ways. Financially it is a boon to the doctors who perform the tests. Doctors who place stents in blocked arteries, put people on dialysis, and who cure NPH all are paid well for their efforts. I once worked with a gastroenterologist who performed ten or more colonoscopies every morning, in many of which he did not visualize the entire colon for logistical reasons such as a poor colon prep. His patients called him very thorough, and he was paid quite well for those tests. Most gastroenterologists I have known are far more scrupulous, but they are still paid more to perform a test than to say no. And patients often prefer a thorough doctor who will say yes.

Medicare enables patients to be tested as often as they wish, by as many doctors and "experts" they choose to see. Regardless of the need, Medicare will pay as long as we can provide a diagnosis, and that is often the easiest road for doctors and patients to take. Especially with my frail dementia patients, I frequently will offer less thorough advice, such as to increase exercise, eat more protein and fruits, and get out of the apartment and socialize with people. But these solutions reek of surrender. Medicare will not pay for my patient to join a gym and have a personal trainer and nutritional counseling, and it will not finance day care for those with dementia so they can be more active and social. It will also not finance palliative care if they are not near death. This may include home health support, various types of medical equipment, and alternatives to hospitalization, all of which are relatively inexpensive and medically effective while achieving high patient satisfaction. But it will pay for tests and procedures, and it will pay for a patient's and family's unending quest to delve into aging's many unfortunate manifestations of decline, despite the high cost and limited utility of such a thorough approach.

Tests and procedures, when not prudently ordered, are dangerous because they help perpetuate the illusion that we can reverse aging by looking hard enough. Not only is such magical thinking endemic in our society, but it is one fully endorsed by Medicare itself. Medicare rewards doctors who test, and it rewards patients who undergo tests, because tests lead to diagnoses, and everything Medicare ultimately pays for is diagnosis driven. Tests often are necessary, if conducted under the umbrella of common sense and reason. But very often in the elderly they are not helpful and are potentially harmful. Yet that does not curb their excessive use.

While Medicare seeks solutions to save itself from financial collapse by forcing doctors to squander time and effort adhering to quality-care protocols that are of unproven value, it does not place the same standards on its own willingness to pay for tests and procedures that are frequently needless or even harmful. The fact, as we have discussed, that 25 percent of Medicare's total budget is spent in the last weeks of someone's life, paying for tests and procedures in the hope of reversing the ravages of age without there being any meaningful hope of recovery, is a testament to the futility of Medicare's priorities and payment model. It is also a manifestation of the increasingly specialized medical society in which Medicare now exists, as we will explore in the next chapter.

3

EXCESSIVE SPECIALIZATION, EXPECTATION, AND LITIGATION

What's absolutely certain is that we don't need more specialists,
but we do need more generalists.

SHANNON BROWNLEE, *Overtreated*

With the explosion of medicines, tests, and procedures that probe and promise to repair every bothersome symptom or clinical abnormality that may riddle an elderly body has emerged the concept of specialization. At the dawn of Medicare most elderly patients were cared for by their trusted primary-care doctors, rarely needing to see any other health-care practitioners. But now that scenario has reversed. The United States trains and retains more specialist doctors than primary-care doctors, and patients see specialists with increasing frequency. Older patients often are being treated as a series of conditions and diseases, each one confronted independently of the whole person, and each one deserving of the most rigorous attention.

In an excellent article in *The New Yorker*, physician-author Atul Gawande defines a concept called "low-value care." This occurs when doctors order tests and treatments that have been determined to be either ineffective or actually harmful. A group of researchers compiled a list of twenty-six such tests, and found that in a single year 25 to 42 percent of Medicare patients received at least one of them.[1]

Many of these tests we have discussed already, from stents to MRIs to EKGs. They have become commonplace in our medical landscape, the very epitome of thorough. They also demonstrate why a specialized medical society, one that focuses on finding and fixing everything rather than trying to help people in a more holistic way, has led us down such a precarious road.

Specialization is a concept based on two essential assumptions. First is the idea that it is best to treat each medical problem independently and aggressively to achieve maximal outcome, typically by an expert in that domain. Such thinking promotes the notion that by fixing numbers, determining precise scientific causes of ailments, and then repairing all that is wrong, our patients will be healthier. Viewing every ailment and condition under a myopic lens allows the doctor to concentrate on that problem and to better manage it. This is compartmentalization of care. Under such a model, we can tackle problems without regard to how they may impact other conditions in the body, because our focus is only on that one condition. For instance, we can assault blood pressure without concerning ourselves with how our treatment may influence falls, fatigue, kidney function, bladder incontinence, and quality of life; those are not within the purview of the blood-pressure number and can be handled at another time or by another doctor.

The second assumption flows from the first. With specialized care, we do not have to accept the inevitability of aging, but rather with a directed purpose can reveal what is causing the many symptoms and conditions that emerge as people age and then effectively treat them. In other words, specialization assumes that if we ask why each problem is occurring and point our efforts to resolving the cause of the problem, then we can fix the problem and improve outcome. Memory loss, for example, is not a foregone conclusion with aging. There are a plethora of tests that can be conducted, experts to be consulted, drugs and treatments to try. Typically we can even define the cause of the memory loss more precisely and scientifically. Dementia is too vague a term; with enough testing and probing we can ascertain the precise form of dementia, and possibly even discover some root causes and novel treatments.

When one approach to treatment fails, there is likely another doctor, another test, another drug that may nudge us in a more promising direction. Specialization raises our expectations and encourages us to never give up, because somewhere out there is a reason and resolution if we just push hard enough.

Specialization runs counter to the idea of palliative care. In a palliative model, especially when directed toward our oldest patients, we ask questions and probe for answers only if the resolution can provide a high likelihood of improved outcome for the patient as a whole. For instance, with memory loss, we may do a few basic tests that can elucidate easily treatable causes of dementia, and even try some medicines for a brief period if they produce clinically meaningful improvement and lack side effects, but otherwise we will accept the memory loss, not feel obligated to further label it if such precise definitions do not facilitate better treatments, and then work with patient and family to manage it. With hypertension we will treat blood pressure only until the medicines instigate significant side effects, or until they interfere with other problems or symptoms exhibited by our patient, perhaps being more aggressive if the elevated pressure is imparting a clinically important risk to our patient, such as a stroke risk in someone who has had several strokes or a risk of hemorrhage in the eye. We are not concerned with sporadic elevations in blood pressure, since that scenario has a small absolute risk of impacting our patient's life, while the treatment may have adverse effects. There is an underlying assumption in palliation that aggressive testing and treatment of chronic conditions and numbers will likely not impact the overall outcome of survival in the majority of our elderly patients, and should be primarily done to help our patients feel and function better. That is the very antithesis of a specialized model.

Medicare encourages specialization in several ways. Most fundamentally, it pays for specialized treatment without hesitation. If you want to see ten specialists and travel from one medical center to another, there is no limitation imposed by Medicare; all of it will be paid, no referral or permission needed. If your new neurologist wants another brain MRI, even though your primary-care doctor ordered one a week ago, then Medicare will pay, no questions asked. And if then you travel to a medical center where another team of doctors wants to repeat the test again, as well as several others, regardless of whether those tests or consultations have any likelihood of impacting treatment, then those too will be paid for. But Medicare is much less willing to pay for palliation. While obtaining a few MRIs, an annual carotid ultrasound, an EEG, several pages of blood tests, three consults, and some medication trials is all smiled upon by Medicare, at a cost to the taxpayer of many thousands of dollars and with the potential peril of causing side effects and unnecessary interventions, treating the dementia with physical exercise in a gym, brain programs such as luminosity, a few days a week in a day-care center, and even some home health aides to provide companionship and to help alleviate caregiver stress are not paid for at all by Medicare. We can search and test interminably under Medicare's umbrella, with cost and outcome being inconsequential, but we cannot manage the problem, even if such management is both effective and economical. In fact, partially due to the changes from the Affordable Care Act, even the act of helping patients to get a simple wheelchair requires an act of God, pages of papers, and criteria often impossible to satisfy, yet that wheelchair may allow a person with dementia to get out of the house, be less agitated, and avoid expensive and debilitating hospitalization at a tiny cost.

Medicare also encourages specialization by promoting the dramatic explosion of specialty care within our medical landscape. As we will discuss, specialists get paid far more than primary-care doctors under Medicare's reimbursement system, and those who perform procedures are remunerated even more generously, thus incentivizing a model of procedure-oriented specialization that has become common in our geriatric universe and that is very costly to the system without producing improved outcomes. Because of the financial gap between primary care and specialty care in this country, we have a significant shortage of generalist doctors and an abundance of specialists.

My grandmother, who had virtually no serious medical problems, saw multiple specialists and no primary-care doctor. Medicare allowed unfettered access to specialty care, even though she enjoyed good health. She urinated too much, so she saw a urologist. She had pain, so she saw an orthopedist and a rheumatologist. She had the shakes, so she saw a neurologist. She could not see and hear well, so she saw an ophthalmologist and otolaryngologist. She continued seeing my grandfather's cardiologist even though she had no heart problems. And I think she saw a gastroenterologist for a little icing on the cake. What struck me as a doctor in training was watching her march to her squadron of specialists with such regularity that those visits became a large part of her life. And when I asked her why she did not have a primary-care doctor, my ninety-year-old grandmother bluntly told me that it would be senseless to see one doctor who knew a little about everything when she could see experts in every field.

The visits did not come without a price. Forget the thousands of dollars Medicare paid for her unnecessary foray into the world of thorough medicine, and the fact she had to financially contribute nothing at all. More significantly, she was given inappropriate medicines on several occasions that directly led to harm and to hospitalization, and she was exposed to potentially dangerous tests and drug interactions. Her neurologist thought she might have Parkinson's (which even as a medical student I knew she did not have), and he started her on a medicine to cure it, a medicine that made her hallucinate. She called my father one night and told him that there were birds in her room having a party. Off she went to the hospital. Several months later her urologist gave her the same medicine, with the same results, landing her back in the hospital. In the end, her death was triggered by a medicine that she should have never received, given to her by a specialist who was concerned about helping the pain in her back but who was not wise enough to know how his treatment would impact the rest of her body. And in the end, too, she spent the last few days of her life in the intensive care unit of a hospital at a cost of thousands of dollars a day, and were it not for the strength and wisdom of her son—my father—she could well have been there far longer with an outcome that in no way would have been good.

Specialists

Specialists are part of the reason that the US medical system is one of the best in the world when it comes to complex and serious medical problems. The United States boasts some of the best-trained and capable specialists of every discipline, and I am always thankful there is a willing specialist available when I need one for my patients. In my experience most specialists are superb doctors who happen to be trained to master a small set of problems. Someone who is very ill, or has a medical problem requiring a procedure or a specific expertise, often does need specialty care.

The problem with specialization in the elderly is not related to very ill patients who need intense procedure-oriented care. Rather, it occurs when patients have fairly simple and straightforward problems, such as diabetes or hypertension or stable heart disease, problems that can be easily managed by a primary-care physician. In our society, with so many specialists and so few primary-care doctors, patients with simple chronic issues often see specialists frequently, leading often to redundant care and narrowly focused care for each individual problem. Sometimes such care is prompted by patients themselves, who want experts for each of their ailments, sometimes by busy primary-care doctors who look to get some help in managing some of their elderly patient's litany of problems. All of this is paid for by Medicare.

In my opinion, the most salient purpose of specialty care is to have experts treat people with complex problems, not to follow uncomplicated chronic ailments. Consequently, I have seen many specialists refer simple problems back to the primary-care doctors, while turning away older patients who request colonoscopies, stress tests, and chemotherapy. I have seen many generalists, however, buy into the specialized model of care, referring patients to specialists for every one of their ailments, and even tossing medicines and tests at older patients every time one of them complains about a symptom or exhibits an errant number. Specialization is a mindset, a manifestation of the concept of thorough, a need to fix numbers and nuisances one organ at a time without having to contend with the broader ramifications that treatment triggers. Most specialists I know would prefer to see more complicated patients rather than the deluge of routine visits that our specialized society sends their way.

When people are young and healthy they develop more unusual and severe diseases that require intensive management by specialists. In fact, young people who do get sick rarely have to see primary-care physicians. But when they are older, and every organ begins to deteriorate simultaneously, when function and memory declines, and when quality of life is more impacted by medical intervention than duration of life is, then a more palliative and holistic approach makes sense for the management of chronic medical problems. Specialization of care removes one problem from the rest of the body. So while specialized doctors may insist that LDL cholesterol be kept below 70 as some clinical guidelines suggest (or under 100 as Medicare's quality indicators cite as good care), pounding their patients with statins, and insist that Coumadin levels in patients with A-fib remain strictly within the parameters elucidated by clinical guidelines, ordering frequent lab checks and dose changes to prevent a stroke, and push patients' blood sugars down with more and more medicines, having patients check their finger-stick sugars incessantly, they need not be concerned about the patient's lethargy and incontinence and osteoporosis and leg weakness and depression and dizziness and memory loss and stress, some of which are made worse by the treatments they prescribe. They can concentrate all their efforts on a problem or two and "fix" those problems intensely, even if their patients become weaker and more confused as a result.

As a generalist, I have to take a broader view. I cannot worry about whether a patient's LDL cholesterol falls into some preordained range, because when it is juxtaposed against all his other problems and concerns, I know that such fine tuning will achieve no useful clinical outcome, may limit my ability to treat bigger problems that impact the patient, and can often cause side effects that impair quality of life and function. I also know that if I grapple with every minor numerical deviation and problem, despite what the clinical guidelines or a few narrow studies of relative risk suggest, I will flood my patient with medicines, test him excessively, and shift the patient's focus away from what may be more important. So for my patient with high LDL, even though he may have had a heart attack ten years ago and the data demands that he needs to be on a statin (with its impressive relative risk reduction but negligible absolute risk reduction), I may suggest he get off his cholesterol medicine if he has leg weakness and confusion (possible side effects of the drugs), advising him that we no longer check his cholesterol or worry about it.

My goal as a generalist is to prioritize problems and not focus on number fixing and on marginal interventions that will not help my patients remain happy, active, and independent and that may increase side effects. It is to present patients with well-explained options and help them decide what is best for them. When my patients have fourteen problems, and come to me on twenty medicines, I can more globally see how fixing one problem impairs another, and how so many pills with so many interactions and untoward side effects do not move my patient toward any beneficial outcome despite an improvement in the numbers. After discussing it with patients or their families, I am often able to keep my patients away from tests and procedures that may open up more cans of worms and reveal problems that are dormant in their bodies and are best left alone. I try to focus more attention on how they are doing now and how they can improve their health through exercise, diet, and socialization. For older patients, trying to extend life and erase problems through thorough intensive medical care is not a goal that can often be realistically achieved, and when confronted with everything at once, we generalists can grasp that reality and work with it. We are not against medical intervention, but we are very careful to ensure that what we do has purpose.

Unfortunately, what we generalists often inherit are patients bouncing from doctor to doctor, on a multitude of medicines and undergoing copious procedures, with no one doctor able to treat the patients as a whole or to convince them that backing off may help them feel better.

The Ramifications of Specialization

Specialized care can have adverse consequences for our elderly. The bloated supply of specialists in our country may actually be impairing the health of our elderly, often because there are just not enough primary-care doctors.[2] In areas with fewer primary-care doctors compared to specialists, older people fare worse in their treatment of cancer, stroke, coronary artery disease, and overall death rate.[3] Overall, in parts of the country with an overabundance of specialization, there is a substantial increase in cost of care, hospitalization, and doctor visits without any significant improvement in outcome.[4] Using Medicare data, Fisher and Wennberg from Dartmouth show that in highly specialized areas of the country older people are less healthy and they die earlier despite similar risk factors. They estimate that 30,000 elderly Americans die each year due to excessive care.[5] Also, regions with more specialists report more medical errors, especially in the hospital.[6] Again, this is not the fault of specialists, but rather of specialization.

Mrs. W. had dementia. We ascertained that fact, put her through some basic tests, and even tried a dementia medicine that I stopped because of side effects. Mrs. W.'s daughter wanted to be aggressive in assaulting the dementia and not let it fester and progress. She had read a lot on the

Internet about treatments that could slow or reverse the flow of the disease, and she could not understand why I was being so lackadaisical in treating her mother's horrible memory loss. I suggested a more holistic approach: more social interaction perhaps through a day-care program, more exercise, and the implementation of strategies to help curb untoward behavioral outbursts. But Mrs. W.'s daughter felt that that was giving up. Mrs. W. saw a neurologist, who ordered more extensive tests, repeating some I had already done, and put her on more drugs. Now the dementia was labeled as frontal lobe dementia, something her daughter felt obligated to explain to me, as if I had been unable to arrive at her mom's true diagnosis. She regularly brought her mother to the neurologist, who by the daughter's own account was a leader in his field, a dementia expert, and a professor at a major academic institution. She also brought her mother to various other specialists regularly. She continued to see me and give me the reports from those more skilled physicians. Her mom was now on a large amount of medicines. She became sick frequently, possibly from the medicines, possibly from stress, possibly from other conditions that consumed her aging body. These illnesses often drove her to the hospital, where more tests were conducted to solve each problem that popped up one after another, leading to trips to more specialists and to more tests and more medicines. When her mom's mental decline became more accentuated, the daughter became disenchanted with her formerly brilliant neurologist and dragged her to yet another neurologist, and started dabbling in alternative medicines and herbal pills about which she became an expert from studying the Internet and taped episodes of Dr. Oz. Eventually Mrs. W. faded from my practice; I think her daughter found another primary-care physician, or perhaps none at all, or maybe had to place her in a nursing home. The search for a cure through specialization did not help Mrs. W.; in fact, to me, it hampered a more reasonable approach to dementia that may have provided Mrs. W. and her daughter a higher quality of life.

The search for a dementia cure is irresistible for many patients and families. We have discussed already the futility of finding a reversible cause of dementia even with extensive testing, and we talked about the very modest impact that dementia drugs have on those who suffer from dementia, often producing no clinically significant functional improvement, which persists only for a few months in a minority of patients, and that can be associated with serious side effects. Still, I have seen specialists order an abundance of tests, prescribe drugs at high doses and in multiple combinations, and promise that their approach is thorough and effective. Hope often trumps reality as so many of my patients and families pursue a specialized aggressive course that leads nowhere beyond frustration, a course that Medicare finances, that the press applauds, and that the public believes to be thorough and miraculous.

Mrs. A. was in her nineties and loved her many specialists, especially her heart doctor, who was a devoted and personable physician. I never could ascertain why she started seeing him in the first place; she had no cardiac history and disdained medicines. Mrs. A. lived with a high blood pressure for over a decade, if not more; numbers of 230/110 were not uncommon. She felt well and was clearly healthy, going to the gym every morning and socializing with friends most of the day, so I never chased those numbers. But her specialists were uneasy, and incessantly put her on blood pressure medicines, fearing she would otherwise get a stroke. Soon after that, she started fainting and feeling tired. She even went to the hospital on numerous occasions after fainting, where she received more tests and more medicines. She saw a neurologist, who looked for other causes of the dizziness through tests and labs. Somehow, even after she and I talked and we agreed to eliminate her blood pressure medicines, she always landed back on them even though she felt better off of them. She, like many of my patients who see specialists regularly, had annual tests, such as heart tests and blood tests, some of whose results were abnormal, which prompted more testing and treatment. The tests and their results made her nervous, but she continued to pursue whatever her doctors asked of her. And she continued to faint every time she went back on her pressure medicines.

I had another patient recently who was an elderly diabetic on insulin. She felt tired and had several episodes of low blood sugar, causing her to be miserably ill. She checked her sugars frequently, being almost obsessed with the fluctuation of her numbers. I felt her sugars were too low, but her diabetes doctor felt they were too high and continued to prompt her to eat better and take more insulin. Finally I convinced her to try less insulin, and then no insulin, and even to check her sugars less. She felt terribly guilty for doing it, afraid she was letting her diabetic doctor and herself down, and that she might get very ill from her misbehavior, even losing a leg or having a stroke. But she felt better, and her A1C sugar level remained decent, although much higher than her diabetic doctor wanted. She never did tell her sugar doctor about it; it was our little secret.

Another of my patients had worsening kidney function according to the labs, but had no specific abnormalities to indicate he needed dialysis, and was actually feeling quite well. In fact, his labs had been very stable over many years. Still, he was convinced that his kidney doctor believed he was on the verge of dialysis and that any deviation from the doctor's meticulously detailed instructions could cause instant doom to his sickly kidneys. My patient would not even eat a banana or grapefruit, although he very much wanted to. He watched every morsel that entered his mouth, swallowed a handful of minerals and medicines, and, as per instructions of his kidney doctor, made frequent trips to his cardiologist and endocrinologist to assure that his blood pressure and sugar were also tightly controlled lest they precipitate his cascade toward dialysis, even if doing so made him feel worse. Nothing I said could convince my patient that such intensive management was not in fact helping him, when so many others told him that it was. He became consumed by a set of illnesses that were more phantom than real in any meaningful medical context, and his foray into the world of medical specialization certainly detracted from his quality of life without necessarily helping him to be healthier. Still another of my patients had a dialysis shunt put in his arm a year prior because his kidney doctor convinced his wife that dialysis was imminent. The man had severe dementia and exhibited many concerning declines in his function, but his wife now had to worry and fret about dialysis and kidney failure, even though his kidney numbers, while abnormal, had not changed in years. She certainly did not need that extra stress, and it was very unlikely that any kidney intervention would improve either the quality or duration of her husband's life.

Specialization can be lifesaving for acute illness, as we have discussed. But there is very little reason for specialists to follow patients regularly for stable conditions, especially as they age and have so many concomitant medical problems, when the treatment of one issue can worsen something else. Still, many patients appreciate such care, Medicare pays for it without question or referral, and with an abundance of specialists in our society, coupled with the higher revenue that procedure-based medicine generates, it is no wonder that specialization has become the norm for older patients with chronic illness.

The Cost of Specialization

An excellent illustration of specialization and its ramifications relates to skin cancer. We are always being told to inspect our skin and to look out for cancers. Some cancers are deadly (melanoma especially), others are less likely to kill or maim. In my older patients the nonlethal skin cancers (squamous cell and basal cell carcinomas) are fairly ubiquitous, sometimes strewn over their bodies. Years of sun exposure takes its toll. I always inspect my patient's skin but I am rarely alarmed, even if I suspect a cancer, unless the lesion is growing, causing discomfort, or demonstrates worrisome features. But when my patients decide to visit dermatologists, those bumps suddenly take on an urgency and must be excised immediately, sometimes requiring surgical eradication. A recent study estimates that 2.2 million Americans are diagnosed with nonmelanoma skin cancers annually, mostly older people in the Medicare age group. These cancers are typically slow growing and do not impact survival or quality of life. Still, most had the lesions removed, and 20 percent of the older patients reported a significant complication of the procedure, including poor wound healing, numbness, and pain. Still, despite the potential harm and the lack of demonstrable efficacy, it is recommended that all such lesions be removed.[7] Dermatologists are well compensated for their thorough "lifesaving" procedures; Medicare pays the bill, and the lay press promotes the importance of getting regular skin checks to cure those skin cancers. But are our patients better off having been exposed to a surgical procedure with no demonstrable impact on mortality or quality of life, even though most think and are told that their lives were saved and their federally financed insurance will blindly pay?

A recent *New York Times* article from January 2014 explored the explosion of dermatology procedures in this country for what are often nonlethal lesions. The article cites the lucrative nature of skin biopsies for the doctors performing them, and the atmosphere of fear that encourages us all to believe that biopsies and radical skin cancer eradication are essential and lifesaving.[8] The truth of such claims is questionable, skin cancer treatment is likely being overutilized, patients are harmed, and Medicare funds are being needlessly squandered. But nothing is being done to stop the process, and in fact more doctors and patients are buying into this aggressive model of care.

When we examine why Medicare is going broke we do not have to look much beyond the skin. The perception that we should be looking for and eradicating every disease process in our older patients is a myth that is inscribed into the very soul of Medicare itself, as Medicare is focused on finding and fixing diagnoses and numbers rather than helping people age well and feel better. Many Americans understand that Medicare is wasteful, but few are willing to acknowledge from where such waste emanates. Any restriction of unnecessary care is labeled "rationing," and that word has doomed all past attempts at health-care reform.

Lower-back pain is another prime example of how specialization impacts cost of care. Richard Deyo, in his book *Watch Your Back,* looks at the entire industry that has grown up around back pain, one that enriches doctors and institutions, leads of overtreatment and overtesting, and is actually harmful in many cases to the patients exposed to such excessive care.[9] We have discussed the large numbers of unnecessary MRIs ordered for lower-back pain, an expense that does not improve outcome. Many patients also prefer to see lower-back pain "experts" such as chiropractors and orthopedic surgeons. Evidence suggests that people who pursue specialized care for their back pain do not fare any better than people who see their primary-care doctor, but that the cost escalates substantially.[10] In my experience, back-pain experts order more tests and lucrative procedures (such as epidural injections) rather than focusing on more common sense approaches (weight loss, exercise, lifestyle changes) that may ultimately remedy the pain. Of course, patients do not travel to see back-pain experts to be told to lose weight; they want the MRI and epidural injection. Medicare pays for the MRI and injection without batting an eye, but it will not pay for an exercise or weight-loss program. So we certainly cannot blame the specialist or the patient.

That specialists are paid more for each visit and procedure by Medicare than primary-care doctors is an inequity derived by the specialist-dominated American Medical Association Board that recommends payment to CMS, as we will discuss. But some specialists also generate funds indirectly due to the procedure-oriented nature of their work. A recent *New York Times* article looked at the cost of colonoscopy, a procedure that increased in frequency by 50 percent between 2003 and 2009. Although Medicare's direct payment to the specialist (gastroenterologist) who performs the test has dwindled to about $500 per procedure (a procedure that takes about twenty minutes of time), the actual cost to insurance for a colonoscopy is often over $5,000, with wide regional variation. Colonoscopies are billed as surgeries, allowing doctors to charge Medicare for many "incidental" fees that dramatically hike their reimbursement. They also employ anesthesiologists in their surgical suites, something done nowhere else in the world and that has been shown to be unnecessary, but which further escalates the cost. According to the article, anesthesiologists alone earn $1.1 billion each year from providing the unnecessary service.[11]

The lay press, both TV and print, recently lambasted the 2013 government sequester for denying older people necessary chemotherapy. In the sequester all doctors received a 2 percent cut in our Medicare reimbursement, one of many cuts we will be forced to swallow in the coming years. However, several intravenous infusion centers that administer chemotherapy stated publicly that the cut would prevent them from offering chemotherapy to the elderly, with the assumption being that now those elderly would die from such blatant medical neglect. The press ran with the story, and the public ate it up. But no one thought to ask a few important questions. First, were these elderly patients really in need of intensive intravenous chemotherapy? Second, how much were these infusions centers and their specialist doctors earning that a 2 percent cut in reimbursement would financially ruin them? After all, oncologists are some of the most highly paid doctors in the country.

This history of chemotherapy is a cloudy one, and one I do not have time to explore in this book. Suffice it to say that cancer specialists had until recently been paid very well to administer intravenous chemotherapy in their offices rather than prescribing oral treatment. In fact, when oral pills were given, the oncologists not only lost the huge markup they received on the intravenous drugs, but patients now had to pay for medicine; Medicare paid for expensive intravenous treatment but not for cheaper pills.[12] Of course, most patients believe that intensive intravenous treatment is stronger and more effective than pills anyway, so they appreciated the thorough care that the oncologists were rendering. The truth of that statement clearly strays from reality,[13] but in our specialized society truth is rarely powerful enough to trump perception. When Medicare stopped paying doctors directly for intravenous chemotherapy, the proportion of treatment being given as pills increased.[14] Now, though, infusion centers are paid to give the drugs, and they have an incentive to treat intravenously.

Whether the 2 percent sequester cut truly prevented elderly patients from receiving "necessary" medicine is questionable, but the fact that the press did not ask those questions demonstrates the power and penetration of thorough care in our specialized medical world.

The Dearth of Primary Care

Unfortunately for our eighty-five-year-old patients, society is inundated with specialized care and with specialists, while there is a dwindling number of generalists willing to take care of them. The United States has it backward with regard to specialists. I have read that in an ideal medical society there should be at least 50 percent generalists. In this country only 30 percent of doctors practice primary care and the rest are specialists.[15] These numbers continue to dwindle. We train many more specialists than primary-care physicians, and a certain assumption prevails among doctors in training and society at large that specialists sit on a higher perch of the physician ladder than primary-care doctors. To many of my patients, and their families, my job as the primary-care doctor is to coordinate their specialty care, to be a unifying presence. In other words, I exist not to render medical treatment, but rather to oversee the compartmentalized and intensive care that is being conducted within a specialized health-care delivery system.

I remember when I interviewed at a large New York City hospital for medical school with the dean of admissions, and I told him that my interest was in primary care. He said that a school like his did not train primary-care doctors, because any school can train primary-care doctors. At elite institutions they train specialists. I fought with him about it, and argued that his school should be ashamed of itself for not producing the type of doctor most needed in the country, whose job was the most intellectually difficult, even citing the fact that his hospital's own impoverished neighborhood was neglected by the institution because of its specialized mindset. By the time I returned to college a week later, the dean's rejection letter was already in my mailbox. Even the medical school I did attend, which had a reputation for taking care of its impoverished neighborhood, and which produced some of the most prolific primary-care thinkers in the world, sent the vast majority of its graduates to specialist programs.

The result of this trend is a dearth of primary-care physicians and an abundance of specialists. In the medical worlds I have traversed, there seem to be as many cardiologists as internists, and they follow stable patients for simple problems several times a year. They perform procedures such as stress tests and echocardiograms regularly for screening, and control numbers (blood pressure, cholesterol) very tightly. Endocrinologists follow simple diabetics, nephrologists (kidney doctors) follow patients with mild and asymptomatic kidney diseases, neurologists follow patients with stable dementia, and orthopedists follow people with simple arthritis. In all of these cases the specialists perform more tests, control numbers more tightly, and have more of a need to fix problems relevant to their field than do primary-care doctors.[16] When a squadron of specialists follows my patients regularly, I lose control of much of their medical care. But there simply are not enough primary-care doctors out there, so specialty care becomes the norm.

Medical Training and Specialization

Why do so many medical students become specialists? The answer is multifold. First, since so many patients see specialists regularly and are allowed to do so by Medicare and other insurances, there is plenty of work for specialists, and there are more than enough specialty training slots open. Second, since specialty fields are procedure oriented, they are better remunerated and have more of a narrow focus, which is appealing. Many students graduate with tremendous debt and seek a good income, fearing that primary-care salaries will be inadequate to pay back the debt and allow for a decent lifestyle. Third, at least in the view of students, specialists have a more interesting life than general doctors and carry more prestige. Fourth, in the course of their training, students and residents are exposed much more to specialty care than to primary care, since primary-care doctors are less likely to be working in hospitals. Even when primary-care doctors do interact with medical students and residents, they are academic doctors, not the type of doctor most students and residents would ultimately become; there is minimal exposure to purely clinical primary-care physicians. Fifth, many of the patients seen by students and residents in the hospital during the course of their training are either "interesting cases" with highly complex specialty needs, or "boring cases" such as old nursing-home patients who were brought to the hospital for custodial care, the latter being perceived as the purview of the primary-care physicians who had cared for them on the outside.

The dwindling supply of students and residents pursuing primary care has significant ramifications for the health of our elderly and the survivability of Medicare. In US medical schools, substantially fewer students retain interest in primary-care fields compared to what they originally stated at the start of their schooling.[17] Even worse, only about 20 percent of students actually pursue a primary-care field by the end of their training. That compares to 54 percent of students who entered primary care in 1998.[18] Medical schools, which do very little to encourage students to enter primary care, consistently try to exaggerate how many potential primary-care doctors they train without actually encouraging their students to enter primary care.[19] Primary-care residency slots remain unfilled more than others, have the highest level of dissatisfaction among students, and suffer from a perceived lack of prestige.[20] Therefore, it is no surprise that we have a primary-care shortage in this country. The number of doctors who practice primary care dropped from 59 percent in 1949 to 37 percent in 1998,[21] and that number continues to decline. With the many costly and time-consuming reforms being thrust on the laps of primary-care doctors by the ACA and Medicare, large numbers of practicing doctors are either retiring, refusing to accept Medicare, or becoming concierge practices that take no insurance at all. This is only exacerbating our primary-care shortage, and it is likely to get worse.

In my own experience as a medical student and medical resident, I had the good fortune to be exposed to a wealth of wonderful primary-care thinkers. But in New York most of the students turned their backs on primary-care fields, and very few of us pursued that route. Even those who accepted residencies in internal medicine explicitly stated that they intended to seek further training as cardiologists or gastroenterologists, two of the most highly reimbursed specialties at the time. My residency training was unique in that many primary-care thinkers taught us, but even there less than a third of our class left training to practice primary care, a number that is far higher than the national average. According to the doctors who still work there, only a handful enter primary care now. I remember in our first week of residency a fellow resident approached me and my wife. She asked us what we were planning to do after training. I told her primary care, and she smirked. My wife told her maybe something like gastroenterology or endocrinology. The woman smiled at my wife, "Good for you," she said. "Those are much better choices." That woman became our chief resident and ultimately a cardiologist, and her view is very common among those who train in my field. Most think you have to be insane to become a primary-care doctor. Both my wife and I practice primary care, and we enjoy our jobs immensely. But without a doubt I am among the few who still would enter primary care if given the choice today.

Primary-care doctors earn far less than specialists. The salary discrepancy in medical fields is not something the free market determines. If that were the case, why would anesthesiologists make substantially more money than some surgeons who actually operate?[22] Patients spend time and effort to pick out their surgeons, and the ultimate outcome of their operation is largely in their surgeon's hands. Anesthesiologists certainly play an important role in the surgery, as do nurses and other ancillary staff, but patients do not chose them or even give much thought to what they do. In the free market, they likely would pay a surgeon far more than an anesthesiologist. In most cases, patients do not have any impact on or knowledge of what any of their doctors earn.

The choice of what a doctor earns is in the hands of CMS. Medicare sets rates, and then most other insurances follow suit. If I earn $100 for seeing a patient in the office and a cardiologist earns $150 for a visit and a dermatologist earns $200 to cut off a mole, those charges are dictated directly by CMS. We as physicians cannot charge any more or less than what CMS dictates, and patient preference and the free market have no role.

At a 2013 AMDA conference (American Medical Directors Association or Society for Post Acute and Long-Term Care Medicine) we heard a talk by Paul McGann from CMS about new changes in Medicare, and several people in the audience asked why CMS did not work harder to achieve some reimbursement parity among doctors. He told us that in fact CMS had delegated the determination of reimbursement rates to the AMA (American Medical Association) as a way of appeasing doctors, and it was that agency that had not done anything to ameliorate the salary discrepancies.[23] The Relative Value Scale Update Committee (RUC) is a thirty-one-physician committee in the AMA that recommends what CMS will pay for visits and procedures. The committee is specialist dominated, and thus primary-care doctors have little voice.[24] The committee meets every year to derive income formulas, basing much of its calculation on estimates of how much physician time a procedure or visit requires. But, as the *Washington Post* revealed, those time estimates are greatly exaggerated for specialty procedures. Also, since the members of the committee are largely appointed by specialist societies, "the problem arises from giving the AMA and specialty societies too much influence over physician pay."[25] Given that only a minority of doctors belong to the AMA, and that virtually no primary-care doctors are part of the organization, it is not surprising that it has done nothing to fix this crucial problem. What is surprising is that CMS, which is incessantly trumpeting the need for more primary-care doctors in any sensible medical-reform model, has done nothing to remedy the ultimate barrier to people actually pursuing primary-care fields: pay inequity. By one report the average orthopedist earns $421,000, cardiologist $376,000, anesthesiologist $358,000, gastroenterologist $370,000, and primary-care internist $196,000.[26] By any calculation, primary-care doctors are earning approximately half what other specialists make. CMS has given primary-care doctors a 10 percent bonus on all Medicare billing for the past few years, but as of January 2016 that has been slated to be eliminated, essentially cutting primary-care income and pushing primary-care doctors even deeper into the physician salary basement. Primary-care doctors have had tremendous increases in overhead and nonreimbursed workload due to the reforms of the ACA and Medicare, and now we are going to be asked to pay for those expenses with a lower Medicare reimbursement. It is difficult to understand how such a decision to cut the 10 percent "bonus" will ameliorate our primary-care crisis and allow primary-care doctors the time and resources to care for our patients appropriately.

Because primary-care doctors do not have a lobbying organization, while most other specialties do, no one is pushing very hard to create an environment in primary care that would attract new recruits. That is why there is no perceivable end to our specialized society. Even if Medicare changed its rules and dissuaded older patients from following a specialized path in pursuit of their health, there simply would not be enough primary-care doctors around to take up the slack.

The Problem with Heightened Expectations
in a Specialized Society

Heightened expectations often drive specialized care, because many patients believe that thorough diagnosis and treatment is the best way to attack and defeat medical decline. There is hardly a patient who has received a stent who does not credit his cardiologist for saving his life, proclaiming that no other course of care would have saved him. Patients are similarly indebted to the endocrinologist who treats their diabetes, or the neurologist who put them on the lifesaving Alzheimer's drug after conducting thorough testing, or the nephrologist who is keeping a close eye on their kidney function and repairing every possible errant number that if left unchecked would kill them, or even who puts them on dialysis.

But when expectations escalate, then poor outcomes are viewed not as part of the inevitable decline that comes with aging, but rather as failure. People become obsessed with looking for and fixing everything, something they have come to believe is achievable. That is the natural consequence of our specialized society. Unlike in the case of Mrs. A., who I described in the introduction, the success of medical intervention is no longer measured by happiness and quality, but rather by tests and numbers and life expectancy. Mom may be happy, but she is not well, her medical conditions are not adequately controlled, and we are going to do whatever it takes to ascertain why. And when Mom declines further, we all wonder how that can possibly happen, even as experts repair one leak after another in her fragile body, when they fix her numbers and order more tests. The problem is never viewed as being related to aging itself, or even ascribed to the faulty repair work being done, but rather is regarded as a sign of even more fixable problems that are amenable to still more repairs as long as we fight hard enough to identify the salient issues. Specialization does not accept defeat. Specialization pushes everyone to keep digging deeper into elderly bodies, keep pouring in drugs and tests, keep monitoring every possible number, without any regard to quality. It is the very antithesis of a palliative approach to care. And it leads to an expectation that adverse outcomes are not acceptable.

I found it fascinating that in my ACO, which is a new Medicare program designed to save money that we will discuss later, one of the quality indicators on which I will be graded, and on which my monetary bonus may be calculated, is access of my Medicare patients to specialists. Even as they innovate to cut costs and provide quality care, Medicare is rewarding doctors who encourage their elderly patients to pursue specialized care. Medicare does not seem concerned that our specialized medical society may be having an adverse impact on the health of older Americans and on the rapidly increasing cost of care. Somehow, it has missed the boat on that one.

Lawyers

One untoward consequence of our specialized society and its heightened expectations is a belief by Americans in the invincibility of the health-care delivery system. If an illness is not cured, if an untoward medical outcome occurs, if the perils of aging cannot be reversed, then certainly someone has to be at fault. After all, with so much technology, so many promises, such well-trained experts who have the most advanced tools at their disposal, why should any of our older citizens have to endure medical declines? When bad outcomes do occur, often a finger is pointed and someone is blamed. Such thinking is what triggers the fear of malpractice among many in the medical community, a fear that instigates a posture of defensive medicine leading to even more aggressive care and higher societal costs.

Is malpractice really as bad as doctors think? My father, who is a lawyer, often debunks the myth of malpractice. He claims that no lawyer in his right mind would take a case that does not have merit, because the cost of researching and litigating such a case would far exceed any potential payment. Much of the literature would agree.[27] Also, medical errors do occur, and patients and their families need a reasonable mechanism to be compensated for egregious mistakes. Thus, in some cases, medical malpractice litigation can be justified.

And yet, malpractice, or the fear of malpractice, impacts everything we do. Not just what we do as doctors, but what patients think. How facilities and nurses act. And how families interact with the medical system. As long as malpractice remains an incessant threat, it will be an excuse used by everyone in the medical establishment to pursue a course of aggressive medical care.[28] The line "I'm ordering those tests so I'm not sued" is heard regularly from the mouths of doctors. Even when not spoken, it is often thought.

Several studies have demonstrated a correlation between the degree of malpractice fear experienced by a doctor and his/her likelihood of ordering more tests and procedures.[29] The same phenomenon occurs when physicians have read about a lawsuit or know of doctors who are sued.[30] Such "defensive medicine" leads doctors to practice aggressive medical care despite the fact that they know other more conservative approaches are medically acceptable.[31] And while studies suggest that the threat of malpractice itself does not diminish quality of care,[32] the fear of malpractice certainly exacerbates a costly and dangerous medical ethos that further promotes a "thorough" approach to care.

Who could think otherwise given the omnipresent threat of suit? The TVs are flooded with commercials showing enterprising lawyers pleading for you to call them if you have any adverse outcomes. It may be birth trauma. It may be a symptom that was missed. It may be related to using a particular drug or not diagnosing a condition. Or it may be the vague crime of nursing home negligence, as we will discuss later.

Over a typical forty-year career, a physician will be involved with an open, unresolved malpractice claim 11 percent of the time, which amounts to 50.7 months on average.[33] Most doctors often know someone being sued or have read about high-profile cases, so the threat of legal action, whether real or imagined, sits heavily on us when we make clinical decisions. I am one of those doctors.

During my office hours one day, an official-looking person (I thought he was a policeman) stood outside my exam room door. When I walked out, he handed me a letter. "Dr. Lazris, I am serving you with a summons." It was one of the most demeaning and frightening moments of my professional career. I could only wonder what I may have done. Many possible incidents flooded my brain. Meanwhile, the patients standing in the office peered at me as though I had done something very wrong. Word soon reached my other patients too. Dr. Lazris was served a summons.

I made a few calls and was given the number of a lawyer, who I was told would be representing me. I was also given the name of the patient whose daughter was initiating the legal action. Her mother had actually been one of my favorite patients, and she had a daughter with whom I got along well. She was ninety-eight years old, had moved to the nursing home where I worked because of worsening dementia, frailty, and poor balance, and then had moved to another nursing home facility for reasons I believed were related to her being too far from her daughter, and at that point I lost contact with her. She did very well in the original nursing home, but her daughter did not like it at all. She was very upset about losing control over her mom's care. She felt her mom was not given enough attention, was not given her medicines properly, and was treated with neglect. She complained to me about it several times, and on each occasion I did what I could to help alleviate the daughter's fears. In fact, despite her daughter's concerns, my patient thrived in the nursing home, and was usually happy and healthy.

I requested her chart from medical records, and I dug through it for many hours. I still could not conceive of what I had done wrong. My lawyer called, and offered only vague answers. He was pleasant, and he said I should not worry. We set up a time to meet in about a week. I canceled all my patients for that day, the first of many times I would have to halt my clinical duties to pursue this frustrating case.

I traveled to Baltimore, to a large building where my lawyer had a beautiful office high above the city. He explained the case to me. Apparently the patient had developed a cough. She was treated with Robitussin by a nurse practitioner who worked at the nursing home, although not as my employee. A few days after that, the patient's cough had not resolved, although she was otherwise well. The nurse practitioner then started antibiotics. The patient became weak for a few days and ate poorly. At some point during this period the daughter had called me, and I saw the patient. By that time she was recovering, and soon after was her usual self. But the daughter claimed that delay in treatment for bronchitis had caused her mom to decline to the point that she was now restricted to a wheelchair.

I looked at my lawyer, both confused and scared. There was no case here. Nothing went wrong. This was a ninety-eight-year-old woman who was treated properly for a common infection. She had no adverse outcome. In fact, I later learned that she lived to almost a hundred. I told him that this case has to be dismissed.

"It doesn't work that way," he told me.

My lawyer informed me that an expert witness—a doctor hired by the prosecuting attorney—had reviewed the case and found that there were issues of negligence. I looked over his case and found it to be medically unsound in every way. My lawyer told me to take notes on the expert's accusations and prepare counterarguments. More work, more stress.

Frivolous malpractice cases such as mine cannot succeed without willing doctors who are paid well to create a plausible argument against the doctor being sued. Many experts are retained by lawyers when they feed the lawyers what they request. So all the incentive for these "experts" is to agree with the lawyer's case and find evidence to support it.[34] The "expert witness for hire" business is a lucrative and thriving industry among physicians. Many doctors advertise their services in legal magazines, many obtain a large portion of their income from helping lawyers.[35] No expert has to ground their claims in the concrete block of truth or standard of care. Some provide "dishonest or medically unjustified testimony due largely to the lucrative nature of expert testimony." Judges do not balk at such practice; they allow all testimony in their courts, leaving it to the plaintiff's "expert" to debunk the defense's "expert," and for the jury to ascertain which expert's claims are legitimate.[36] Certainly the expert who had scripted the case against me seemed to have no knowledge of geriatric medicine, and his arguments fell apart quickly.

Nonetheless, the case continued. I went for depositions, taking more time off from work. Letters back and forth. More accusations for me to challenge. And then something happened, something that shocked me more than anything else that transpired during this case, and something that ended the case for good.

My lawyer called me. He told me that the patient's daughter just had her deposition, the very daughter who had brought the case against me. And in the deposition she said that the only good thing that happened during her mother's time at the nursing home was her relationship with Dr. Lazris. She made it very clear that I had done nothing wrong.

"That has to end this case!" I insisted to my lawyer.

And in fact, by that afternoon, the case against me was dismissed.

Still, to this day, the case haunts me. Not because it replays in my mind, although it does do that, because it reminds me just how broken the system is. But more pragmatically, there is not an application to an insurance company or to a hospital or to a license that I fill out on which I do not have to indicate that I was sued, and then provide a separate explanation about what transpired. It is as though I am scarred by the suit, and I will be for the rest of my professional career. Even though the frivolous case was dismissed, it hangs over me and causes me endless inconvenience and embarrassment.

Malpractice suits are often justified, but frivolous suits breed a culture of aggressive care and heightened expectation that is both counterproductive to older patients and very expensive. The fact remains that as long as malpractice hovers over the medical community in its present unfettered form, it will impact behavior. As with the dogma of specialization that fuels it, malpractice feeds on an assumption ingrained in our culture that adverse outcomes cannot be tolerated and that older patients require the most excessive care possible in an effort to save them; anything short of that is negligence. Such a belief often sends patients to the ultimate institution of aggressive, specialized, and thorough care that exists in our country: the hospital. It is that institution that we will explore next.

4

HOSPITALIZATION

The Pinnacle of Thorough

Most people die in hospitals, tied up with tubes and with their bodies
pumped full of drugs. Yet most would rather die at home and with more
control over the timing and manner of their death.

GEOFF MULGAN, CEO, National Endowment for
Science Technology and the Arts (UK)

The ultimate ramification of specialization, of the need to thoroughly
defeat aging by righting every unearthed ailment and flooding the body
with pills, tests, and procedures, is hospitalization. If specialty care is
needed to address each problem that arises, then hospital level of care is
necessary when those problems become severe. In the hospital, patients
can receive intensive treatment, all the necessary tests and procedures, the
strongest medicines, and access to every form of specialty care. Hospitals
have saved many of my oldest patients at some point in their lives. Just ask
them or their families, and they will tell you. Recently I had a patient tell
me that if he had come to the hospital only ten minutes later, he would
have died. These are common tales I hear every day. They are visions of
hospital care shared by patients, doctors, and society at large. But if we explore why Medicare is failing, and to where a large chunk of its expenses
are evaporating without improved outcome, we do not have to look much
beyond the hospital.

Especially at a point of desperation, many elderly people and their families, as well as their doctors, believe that only a hospital can provide the needed care to bring a gravely ill person back from the brink of drastic decline. What we will show is that in fact hospitals frequently instigate more harm in the elderly than benefit. But more significantly, the hospital is perceived as a beacon of care not only because of what it is felt to provide, but because no other options exist. As we discussed, Medicare's inception in 1965 came with a caveat: the hospital would remain predominant in the spectrum of care. Few regulations hampered hospital care, and in fact hospitalized care fell under the umbrella of Medicare A, an insurance given to all elderly and disabled people without charge. Medicare pays for hospitals, and because Medicare A is typically easier to access and more generous in its allocation of resources than Medicare B, the hospital is often the least expensive destination for ill patients.

Four million Americans have part A only, which represents 6 percent of all Medicare beneficiaries. Part A requires patients to pay a $1,184 deductible, after which all services are covered for the first sixty days.[1] People with only part A have no choice but to travel to the hospital for all of their care. Ninety percent of elderly Americans also carry a supplemental insurance plan that pays for the hospital deductible and for the 20 percent that Medicare B does not cover, thus making most medical care free after their part B premiums are paid.[2] The small percentage of people with part B and no supplemental insurance likely will find hospital care less expensive to them than care at home, especially if they need many tests and procedures. But even for those with supplemental insurance, Medicare's rules and payment system frequently push reluctant patients into the hospital. The hospital is a mix of good and bad, especially for our oldest patients; frequently the elderly are sent there for poorly conceived reasons or out of financial necessity, and often the end result is poor outcome at high cost.

Medication Errors

As a medical student in New York I worked with resident doctors, who, in teaching hospitals, essentially manage all facets of patient care. A few days before Thanksgiving, when we were all trying to devise strategies to get out early and spend some time at home, our team was caring for two women, both with similar last names. One had diabetes, the other did not. The diabetic woman was old and had dementia, but her big smile and frequent hilarious one-liners kept us all in stitches. The other woman was fairly ill with a drug-related infection. One day we received an urgent lab result that one of the women's sugars had shot up to 600, a very high value. The resident instructed me to give the young woman insulin and to recheck the sugar in a few hours. But when we did check it the next morning, it remained high, and the young woman looked even sicker than before. We then checked a finger-stick sugar, and it showed a very low sugar number, prompting us to give the young woman an infusion of sugar water into her veins. We thought that there was a lab error, and pushed it aside. The next day on routine labs, we again received notice of a high sugar, this time over 800. Again we checked a finger-stick sugar, and it was now normal. A few days passed, and we then saw another sugar, this time it was 1,200. Suddenly my resident realized what was going on. The labs were actually from the older woman whose name was virtually identical to the younger woman's. When we ran to see her and checked her finger-stick sugar, it was off the charts. She was as happy as can be, and I remember to this day what she said: "Why are all of you coming into the barber shop now? You know I'm next in line. But if you're in a rush, you can go ahead. It's no trouble for me." She died a few hours later, likely from hyperglycemia. But what transpired subsequently inflicted a permanent scar on my medical psyche. As we all feared the consequences of our mistake, the deceased patient's brother came to the hospital bearing a large box of candies. He handed the box to us. "Thank you so much for taking care of my sister," he said with a tear in his eye. "I know she was too sick to be saved by you people, but you gave her the best care she could have got, and the family appreciates all that you did for her." We said nothing. In retrospect, we easily could have killed both patients with our mistake. But instead of a reprimand, we received candy and a hug.

Throughout my days working in hospitals, rushing through patients about whom I knew very little, paging through lists of medicines and tests and numbers, I did my best to keep on top of all medical issues that emerged. But I cannot even begin to relay how often the wrong medicines were given (such as Dilantin, a seizure medicine, instead of diltiazem, a blood pressure medicine), important medicines were overlooked and not given, or even another patient's entire medicine list was inadvertently substituted for my patient's list because of a clerical error, leading my patient to be on completely the wrong drugs, some of which could have been lethal, and to not be on his usual drugs, some of which may have been necessary. I have had patients whose blood pressures plummeted and who were sent to an intensive care unit (ICU) and given the million-dollar workup in search of infection or heart dysfunction, only to find out that they were accidently put on blood pressure medicines that they previously had not taken at home. Sometimes the lists of medicines were derived from past hospital stays, other times they were written down after talking to a family member or a confused patient, sometimes they came from a fax sent by the doctor's office that was either barely legible or inaccurate. Regardless, hospital medication error is something we contend with that is dangerous and difficult to avoid.

Medical mistakes are common in the hospital, especially among the elderly who are often taking many medicines. Such mistakes instigate tremendous morbidity and mortality, making hospital errors the eighth leading cause of death in the country. Each year, 1.3 million hospitalized patients suffer a serious complication from a medical error.[3] Errors occur commonly on hospital admission, but even on discharge, errors occur with similar surprising frequency. As we will discuss, during transition of patients from a hospital to a nursing home, a likely destination for many of the oldest patients in our Medicare community, medicine lists often are severely mangled, and it can require days or weeks to repair the errors and fix any damage that may have been caused.

The Sting of Aggression

Often hospital "mistakes" are of a more insidious nature, resulting from the adrenaline-driven atmosphere that exists within hospital walls. From the time I was a medical student, through my days ward attending in a teaching hospital, I witnessed the deluge of aggression that greets those who enter a hospital's hallowed halls. I remember one day as an attending

I came in and noted that most of my patients were being seen by multiple specialists, all of whom were ordering their own tests and paying close attention to their own organs of interest. I questioned the medical resident, and he told me that as a teaching-hospital resident he felt obligated to have specialists take care of the many chronic problems each patient had, even if the problems were quiescent. Not only did he believe such care to be superior, he also thought it would be educational for the residents on each of the specialty teams to put their hands into the care. How else would they learn?

Even later in my career, I often called in specialists to ease my burden. If a patient was too sick, or I received too many calls from nurses during the day, I made sure to have a cardiologist, a pulmonologist, an infectious disease expert, and even a surgeon look in on my patients to deflect some of my own responsibility. Today I see hospitalist doctors doing the same thing. Hospitalists are doctors hired by the hospital to take care of hospitalized patients, since most of us in primary care are unable logistically to care for our own patients in the hospital. Many hospitalists are very young, just out of residency, with little experience behind them. They do not know their patients well, and in my own estimation very few I have encountered are cognizant of how to care for the elderly. Typically they call in a squadron of specialists, tackling one problem at a time. The end result is specialized, aggressive care.

Mrs. R. went to the hospital for a rapid heartbeat. I usually treat that in my office, and order a little home health so a nurse can keep an eye on the situation, but the cardiologist wanted her in the hospital, and she could not really afford home health aides (which are not paid for by Medicare, while the far more expensive hospital stay is), so there she went. Once there they found she had a little fluid on her lung, so they gave her an intravenous diuretic called Lasix. But they gave her too much. She starting peeing everywhere and getting upset. She also became dehydrated and her blood electrolytes destabilized. Nurses incessantly invaded her room at all hours to draw blood and check vital signs as they carried on conversations outside her room. She started getting delirious. They tied her down and gave her medicine to calm her. She thrashed all the more. Her kidney function worsened from the powerful medications and her inability to eat. They pushed food and fluids on her, and she inadvertently sucked some of the food into her lungs. She developed a raging pneumonia, requiring her to be intubated and hooked up to a breathing machine in an intensive care unit. There she lost blood, developed complications from antibiotics including excessive diarrhea, and required even more aggressive care. She lasted two weeks in the ICU before dying, probably at a cost of over $100,000 paid by Medicare for an outcome that did not have to occur.

Often my older patients are physically tied down in the hospital, are subjected to toxic medicines to calm them down, and become delirious. These are not necessarily people who are ever confused when they are well, but the trauma of the hospital induces it. I remember coming to a medical floor one day to find one of my favorite patients tied down to his bed. He was thrashing and yelling in a way I could have never imagined. I untied him. He had a Foley catheter in his bladder and two IV lines in his arms. I told the nurses to remove all of that and to send him home. They thought I was insane. But within an hour of his arrival home, with his daughter staying with him that night, he was himself again. Hospital delirium is common in the elderly, and the outcomes are not good. Many patients lose function from their delirium and are more likely to develop dementia or have worsening memory subsequent to their hospital stay.[4]

Mrs. G. fell and broke her shoulder. She was already frail, and could not function on her own with a broken shoulder. Ideally she needed either a few hours a day of home health, or a short stay in a rehab unit, both of which were cheap and safe options but not ones she could afford under current Medicare rules. So she went to the hospital, where admission was easily justified by her other medical conditions, some of which had become worse since the fall, including higher blood pressure and a little dehydration. Not only would Medicare pay for the hospital stay, it would pay for up to three months of a rehabilitation stay after hospitalization, something she and her daughter felt would be necessary before she could return home. In order to qualify for paid rehabilitation, though, Mrs. G. had to stay in the hospital at least three nights—a strict Medicare rule. So we agreed to prolong her hospital stay in order to qualify her, something we call "punching our patient's ticket," meaning that we were helping our patients to save some money by keeping them in for three nights. Mrs. G. ultimately did make it to the rehab center, but not until weeks later, and at high personal and financial cost. Her hospital stay nearly destroyed her.

She was given too much pain medicine, developing severe constipation and bowel dysfunction, then a urine infection from her catheter, then diarrhea from the antibiotic used to treat the urine infection and the medicine used to treat her prior constipation, then delirium, and inability to eat, and the need for intravenous fluids, and infections from the intravenous needle sites, and fluid overload, and anemia requiring transfusions, and complications from the transfusions. A half dozen specialists followed her, and she was exposed to tests nearly every day. She had a very thorough hospital stay. I hardly remember all the details, other than how terrible it was. One problem led to another, one treatment to another disaster, until she became a shadow of herself. Medicare did pay for her stay at the hospital and then at the rehabilitation unit, which is all she had wanted, but at a cost of probably a hundred thousand dollars and my patient's soul and vitality.

Mrs. G.'s story is not at all atypical. Older people in the hospital do not fare well. Their bodies are fragile, and treating one problem often instigates another. In the hospital patients are assaulted by aggressive doctors and nurses of every stripe, many of whom are not addressing the problem that brought the patient to the hospital in the first place, but problems that were "discovered" while at the hospital. This leads to more tests, medicines, treatments, and ultimately to more stress, confusion, and complications. And those complications lead to more interventions, which lead to more complications, and so on, until the cascade of failure takes on a life of its own.

A large number of studies demonstrate the poor outcomes caused by hospitalizing elderly people, especially those who are frail and suffering from dementia. The mortality of older adults sent to the hospital is high, both during hospitalization and in the immediate posthospital period. A quarter of hospitalized elders sent from a hospital to a rehabilitation unit are dead within six months despite the extensive resources tapped for their care. Long-term outcomes are much worse.[5] Those hospitalized with advanced dementia have a high short-term mortality, especially when artificially fed.[6] For one of the most common conditions for which the elderly are hospitalized, congestive heart failure, the one-year outcome is abysmal, and the cost of thorough care does not translate into any meaningful results.[7]

Hospitalized elders have significant functional loss after a hospital stay, especially if they become confused in the hospital. This is most pronounced among our frailest elderly and those with dementia.[8] Hospitalization leads to decreased muscle tone, decreased nutritional integrity, and an increase in both urinary incontinence and skin breakdown. Restriction of activity in the hospital accounts for much of this decline, but so too does the avalanche of aggressive care with which the hospital greets oldest patients. Much of the functional loss is irreversible.[9]

Infections

The hospital itself is a brewing caldron of resistant bacteria that can cause terrible infections, even for those who reach only the emergency room.[10] Many of my patients emerge with infections that disable them or take their lives after a hospital stay. It is estimated that preventable infections account for 75,000 deaths a year,[11] and mistakes in the hospital account for 200,000 deaths a year.[12] It is felt that more than two hundred people die of hospital-acquired infections daily, which is as though a plane crashes every day and kills everyone on board. Even one plane crash is front-page news for weeks. Deaths from hospital infections, which occur every day, are barely noticed.

My older, frail patients are particularly vulnerable to the sting of hospital-acquired infections. So many return home or to their long-term-care facilities with massive bouts of diarrhea caused by C. diff, a virulent colon bacteria that flourishes in hospitals and overwhelms the bowels of many older patients, especially if they were exposed to broad-spectrum antibiotics in the hospital. These patients become dehydrated quickly, get confused, develop nutritional depletion, and have significant derangements in their body chemistry. Their functional status declines rapidly and they are unable to participate in rehabilitation. Skin breakdown is common. They are often isolated in their rooms and are unable to leave, being greeted by nurses and doctors wearing gowns and masks, as they sit in a pile of liquid, putrid stool. C. diff is a consequence not only of a hospital stay, but also of even an emergency room visit. We treat it with even more antibiotics, sometimes for weeks, sometimes unsuccessfully. Patients die of C. diff. They physically and mentally decline. And it is more common than people realize.

My patients also return with other resistant bugs such as MRSA, E. coli, and klebsiella. These cause very difficult-to-treat skin infections, urinary tract infections, and even pneumonias. They too lead to decline, more anti-biotics, and isolation. As these superbugs grow in the hospital and latch themselves on to older bodies, they spread beyond the confines of the hospital walls. Like with so many hospital complications, infections occur after discharge and are thus not always ascribed to the hospital stay itself. But the hospital is their immediate cause, and their consequences can be devastating.

The Benefits of Hospitalization?

Given how dangerous hospitals are for the elderly, and how common it is for the elderly to be admitted to hospitals in the United States, there must be a good reason for older patients to be hospitalized. It is common lore that when the elderly are too sick to be cared for at home, when they are met with changes in condition such as worsening memory or dizziness, when they develop serious infections such as pneumonia or potentially dangerous diseases such as heart failure and A-fib, then hospitals are the safest and most sensible places in which to get proper and thorough care. The truth, though, is much more dubious.

I have challenged many doctors to show me a single study that demonstrates the efficacy of hospitalization in the elderly for stroke, pneumonia, change in memory, fainting, small heart attacks, and a wide range of medical problems for which my older patients regularly are admitted. I am still waiting for a response. I have searched the medical literature and found nothing that convinces me of any significant clinical benefit of hospitalization for these conditions that would justify the risk.

In fact, studies show that elderly patients treated in their own beds do as well as or better than those sent to the hospital. Pneumonia is a prime example. In patients who are in nursing homes or who are nursing-home eligible, treatment within the facility or at home affords a better outcome with less functional decline than treatment within the hospital. People die less often, recover more quickly, and are not as prone to delirium as hospitalized patients are.[13] Even more significantly, they are able to stay with nurses and/or family who know them, are in a comfortable environment that is familiar, and are not subjected to the specialized assault that will likely greet them in the hospital.

A congestive heart failure (CHF) study further pounds this fact home. Very few diagnoses are more likely to lead to hospitalization than CHF, a condition where the heart is not functioning properly and the lungs can fill up with fluid. In the hospital such patients are diuresed with medicines that pull fluid out of their lungs. Of course, since they are in the hospital, they are often subjected to multiple tests, specialty visits, new (and often erroneous) medicines, and potential infections. Sometimes they are given too much diuresis, sending them down a road of dehydration, excessive urination, and infection. Almost all of them have a urinary catheter inserted in their bladder and IV lines in their arms, which are more foci of infection and potential delirium. But it is considered standard of care to hospitalize such patients; the only other option would be a more palliative approach whereby they stay at home and are kept comfortable. The basic assumption sewed into palliative care is that such patients, by eschewing aggressive interventions such as hospitalization, are accepting death as the alternative. But research demonstrates just the opposite. With CHF, people live an average of eighty-one days longer with a palliative approach than with standard treatment, including hospitalization. Many other severe illnesses are similarly better treated with palliative care then with aggressive care. In fact, in a Dartmouth study, full-dose palliative care produced better quality of life, decreased depression, and *increased survival* compared to a more standard, aggressive route.[14] Of course, palliative care not only is safer and more compassionate than hospitalization, but it is far less expensive to Medicare and to society.

People treated with a palliative approach are not simply neglected and left to die just because they are not pushed into a hospital and shoved down a bumpy road of thorough intervention. A palliative approach to CHF, for instance, would have as its goal patient comfort, which would therefore aim to reduce the shortness of breath associated with increased fluid retention. Such patients may weigh themselves regularly, be helped with medication and disease management by care coordinators, be offered dietary and exercise counseling, receive periodic visits by home health nurses and physical therapists, and have more regular appointments with their primary-care doctor. The objective is to prevent any exacerbations that may lead to worsening CHF. Since most elderly prefer to stay at home, palliative services can deliver the bulk of their care in the home environment, especially if a patient is considered homebound. The fact that such an approach reflects what most patients request, is less expensive, and leads to better outcomes does not mean that it is feasible. Medicare pays for hospitalization and aggressive management far more than for any meaningful palliative home care, especially for those patients who may require more custodial help.

Many other ill patients would likely benefit by being treated with care and dignity at home instead of in a hospital. Syncope (passing out), strokes, increased confusion, and excessive fatigue are all symptoms that drive many of my patients to the hospital. There is no evidence that hospitalization improves outcomes in any of these conditions, and ample evidence that hospitalization in general is dangerous for elderly patients, as we have discussed. But the natural reflex action when someone faints or becomes confused or exhibits signs of stroke is to push them into a hospital. The latter situation is more nuanced, since obtaining a CT scan for potential stroke victims can help drive treatment depending on whether the patient has a true ischemic stroke or a bleed, but beyond that there is little that the hospital can do to ameliorate the damage done by a stroke in an elderly patient. In my experience, many elderly stroke patients are harmed by the hospital, whether by having their blood pressures pushed too low, or being fed in a way that causes them to aspirate into their lungs, or given fluids and pushed into heart failure. They are also potential victims of resistant infections, medication errors, and hospital-induced delirium.

One significant intervention that can potentially help stroke victims, and that pushes everyone to the hospital as quickly as possible, is TPA (tissue plasminogen activator), or clot-busting medicine. Many of my patients or their families insist that they need to be hospitalized within hours of a potential stroke so they can receive the miracle medicines that dissolve blood clots. But in patients over eighty, according to a study published in 2010, 16 percent of those who received TPA developed a significant brain bleed, and none of the patients who received TPA had improved function compared to standard-care patients after three months.[15]

That is not to say that the hospital is an inappropriate place to go for catastrophic illness requiring intensive care treatment or emergency surgery. But even in those circumstances, in frail elderly patients who have dementia, the hospital may simply make the last days of someone's life more traumatic and extremely expensive. Much end-of-life care occurs in the intensive care unit of a hospital, where expensive and traumatic care leads to no measurable medical benefit for the frail elderly patient.[16] A huge part of Medicare's expenditures is paid for hospital-level care at the end of life, in patients who often are too sick to benefit from such care. The fact that 63 percent of our elderly spend time in the hospital during their last month of life, and that such end-of-life splurging eats up a huge chunk of Medicare's budget without saving life or improving quality,[17] shows that this futile gasp of thorough care within the expensive hospital walls at the end of someone's life makes no medical sense. Doctors and hospitals profit from such aggressive care, but the patient and the system are not quite as fortunate.

Why Is There So Much Hospitalization?

As we have discussed, studies show that a vast majority of elderly people prefer to die at home and not in a hospital, but often their wishes are ignored as the aggressive US medical mentality overrides patient preference.[18] There are many reasons why the hospital has become the destination of choice for those most ill, even those who have explicitly stated that they do not wish to be hospitalized. Some of the fault is more systemic, some is more patient-centric, but all of it is exacerbated by a Medicare system that encourages hospitalization through various means. Although CMS has initiated measures to curb hospital admissions, and although the dangers of hospitalization are well known to most of my patients and their families, Medicare's payment policies continue to push people through the hospital's front door without offering doctors or patients other reasonable alternatives.

Elliott Fisher, who studies regional variation of care within the Medicare population, found that regions of the country with increased numbers of hospital beds and higher specialist concentrations are more likely to hospitalize the elderly. Such regional disparity is not impacted by diagnosis or the extent of illness. These high-spending hospitals will cost Medicare more money per patient because they deliver more intensive care, care that much of the population would consider "thorough." But as Fisher has shown, hospitals that spend the most money in the last six months of someone's life have a 2–6 percent *increase* in death rate compared to low-spending hospitals, irrespective of the degree of medical illness.[19]

But the perception of hospitals is quite different. Just last month a ninety-plus-year-old patient of mine presented to the office with increased confusion and weakness. I suggested to his son that he may have had a stroke, but that hospitalization would not be necessary, since there was nothing we could accomplish in a hospital that would alter his chance of recovery. Instead I suggested he move to a nursing home-rehab unit for a few weeks until he improved. The son agreed at first, but then was persuaded otherwise by those who seemed to know better (friends, family, the Internet), and he sent his dad to the hospital for a more thorough evaluation. In addition, although he did not verbalize it, the hospital would have cost him nothing, while a rehabilitation stay or home care could have cost him many thousands of dollars in out-of-pocket expenses not covered by Medicare. I pleaded with him to get his dad home, but he believed that his dad needed a good looking over before coming home. His dad never did come home. He died in the hospital, from complications created by the hospital, and not from his small stroke. His son did not blame the hospital, and in fact felt just the opposite: he told me that his dad must have been very sick to have died, and it was a good thing that he was in the hospital, which gave him the best chance of living. Such is a misconception that fills the hospital wards with so many elderly people who should not be there.

A few of my patients and their families buy into the notion that the hospital is the best place to go. I have patients who call 911 several times a month, are treated in the emergency room for minor complaints such as elevated blood pressure or dizziness and, several thousand dollars later, after exposure to significant risk, are sent home. Sometimes they are admitted when their story is good enough, and they are more than happy to see a half dozen specialists and have an ample helping of tests in the hope of fixing problems that have been plaguing them for months or years. Medicare pays for the hospital without asking questions. If my patients want to go there every day, Medicare puts up no barriers. And it is typically cheaper for them to sit in the hospital than to find transportation to see their doctor.

But too many of my patients, even the ones who with their families believe in minimalist palliative care, eventually find themselves in the hospital despite expressing firm wishes otherwise. Part of it is fear that, when serious illness rears its ugly head, hospitalization is necessary to avert death. Not knowing what else to do, they call 911. It occurs in a moment of panic, even among people who disdain hospital care. Other families do it out of necessity. They cannot afford to keep their loved one at home, cannot afford a rehabilitation stint, and so resort to the hospital as the one place where their loved one can get care and have that care paid for by Medicare. Why is that? Hospitals provide twenty-four-hour care, paid for by Medicare A, while no part of Medicare pays for adequate care at home.

To obtain sufficient care outside the hospital, patients either have to pay for home health aides, something that Medicare will not reimburse, or spend time in the subacute unit of a nursing home, something for which Medicare A will pay *but only after a three-night stay in a hospital,* as we have discussed. Patients can obtain limited nursing services and rehabilitation at home through Medicare A, but not the custodial care they often need, not the IV fluids if they need that, and often not even the medicines. Not everyone has the financial and human resources to provide home care, especially when Medicare is barely helping, and when a far better reimbursed option exists within the hospital walls.

Ironically, not only is it safer for elderly patients with conditions like pneumonia to stay at home, but it is far less expensive to the health-care system to provide such care at home, even if home care is more expensive for the patients themselves. The cost of treating pneumonia is approximately $10 billion per year, most of which is spent on the elderly, and 92 percent of which is spent on hospital care.[20] In a study of hospital-level in-home services, such as that provided by some VA sites, there was a substantial decrease in cost without decline in treatment quality for those treated at home not only for pneumonia but also for CHF, COPD (chronic obstructive pulmonary disease), and cellulitis.[21] Thus home care would be feasible for the elderly if Medicare paid for it, and it would be both medically beneficial and cost saving. Instead, Medicare's payment system encourages just the opposite.

Medicare similarly nudges doctors like me to send my sick patients to the hospital rather than to arrange home services, because hospitalization is the easiest path for us to take. As Ira Byock observes: "Trying to manage the myriad problems of a chronically ill patient in a busy office can feel like juggling Jell-O on a busy city street corner in a rainstorm. The easiest, safest, and most efficient thing for a doctor to do is to send such acutely ill patients to the hospital."[22] We simply do not have time to jump all the hurdles Medicare puts in the way of doctors who want to help patients stay at home. Arranging home health care is an onerous burden requiring calls and paperwork, and separate calls have to be made to agencies that provide home health aides, if they are even available. Medicines must be called in. Sometimes patients need equipment, such as oxygen or nebulizer machines, each of which requires more calls and paperwork. All this has become even more difficult under new Medicare and ACA rules. Usually these services cannot even start until the following day. My office staff and I have spent countless hours on many occasions trying to arrange services at home, often only to find that the patients cannot afford such services, or the services are not available, or the paperwork must be redone because a portion of it did not comply with regulations. Nothing in the Medicare universe helps us arrange home care; instead, it makes such an endeavor virtually impossible. If we tell our patients to call 911 and go to the hospital, however, our total cost in time is measured in minutes, and our patients feel that we are helping them. Many patients have thanked me for sending them to the hospital just in the nick of time to save their lives. For them and for me, hospitalization is the only feasible route available when they are fairly ill, even though I know that it is not the best route for my patients or our health-care system.

Hospitalization also incentivizes doctors in other ways. Hospital reimbursement is good for doctors, who are expected to see hospitalized patients every day; many of us can see more patients at a higher reimbursement in the hospital than in an office. For specialists and generalists alike, hospital medicine is lucrative. Now many hospitals are hiring their own doctors, presumably to keep some of that money in their own coffers. Hospital monetary arrangements are much too complicated for this book, and many hospitals are always proclaiming that they are on the verge of financial collapse, but their doctors do quite well, as do their CEOs. An August 2012 article in the *Baltimore Sun* showed that most CEOs of Maryland hospitals earn well over $600,000, with thirteen of them earning over a million dollars a year.[23] Certainly, Medicare has been very kind to US hospitals.

Moving in a Sensible Direction

Even as geriatric doctors know that hospital care must be curbed for the good of our patients' health and the survival of Medicare, even as we hope for actual reform that will enable us to treat our patients safely in their homes, which is what so many of us and our patients prefer, we do realize that any assault on hospital care will be met with resistance. That is because hospitals perform a vital role in our society. An American Hospital Association website spells out the economic value of hospitals. They employ over 5.3 million people, are the second-largest source of private sector jobs in the country, spend $320 billion on goods and services, and create over $2 trillion in economic activity. That economic activity creates ripple effects that spur even more jobs and economic growth.[24] Hospitals also are the primary training arena for medical students and residents, are essential for medical research, and perform vital medical services that are both necessary and lifesaving.

Moving a large portion of geriatric care outside the hospital walls will certainly cause these institutions economic injury, even though hospitals will still control a large sector of health-care provision, from trauma care to surgery, obstetrics, and the acute care of heart attacks. But hospitals do not have to abandon geriatric care; they simply have to offer more sensible care. To some extent that is already occurring and, as we will show, some Medicare and ACA reforms are making small attempts to reduce hospitalization among the frail elderly.

ACE (acute care for the elders) units in some hospitals are already accomplishing that goal by providing quality geriatric care at lower cost and with improved outcomes. In an ACE unit, such as one described at Ohio State, older patients considered most at risk for functional decline are identified and treated by an interdisciplinary team expert in geriatric care. There are multiple such units sprouting all over the country.[25] ACE units have been shown to decrease functional decline, decrease the use of restraints, and increase the satisfaction of patients, caregivers, nurses, and doctors. There are also decreased falls, less delirium/confusion, and greater likelihood of a patient being discharged home rather than to a nursing home. There is some evidence that ACE units can decrease length of stay and cost, although these findings are not consistent.[26] Such units allow patients to be discharged from hospitals in better health than occurs in traditional hospital units and with less likelihood that they will be readmitted for the same diagnosis.[27]

Another movement in some hospitals is to establish geriatric emergency rooms that specifically meet the needs of older patients with moderate illness. Holy Cross Hospital in Maryland established the first such unit, and it is popular with both patients and providers of care. In the geriatric ER a team of geriatric doctors, nurse practitioners, nurses, and social workers try to address the more global needs of patients. The rooms are larger and designed for the needs of the elderly, with heated thick mattresses, easily accessed electronics, and increased space for family consultations.[28] A 2007 article describes how such emergency rooms can help meet the very complicated needs of older patients,[29] although no studies to date have demonstrated improved outcome or reduced cost from using geriatric emergency rooms. As with ACE units, the hope in a geriatric ER would be that a patient is given the specific treatment required to help her surmount an acute illness, such as IV fluids if she cannot eat, and then sent home with in-home care. As noted, though, even under the umbrella of its recent reform thrust, Medicare remains stingy with regard to home care, and for patients it is much less costly to receive services at a hospital than at home.

Perhaps the most promising innovation hospitals may consider in caring for the elderly would be the establishment of palliative care programs. The number of such programs has increased nationally. A study of eight hospitals with palliative care services showed that the cost of care was markedly reduced compared to traditional care.[30] Palliative hospital care represents an approach that emphasizes function, satisfaction, and comfort rather than the more aggressive and specialized treatment to which most elderly patients are subjected in hospitals. Diane Meier at Mount Sinai in New York has established a very successful palliative care program using a team approach that we will discuss in greater depth later. Her program increases patient satisfaction, decreases hospitalization, and improves clinical outcome at a much reduced cost to the system. As similar programs proliferate in our hospitals and beyond, our modus operandi can be pushed in a more reasonable direction, and "thorough" will mean comprehensive team-based care that is patient centered and compassionate, rather than protocol-driven care that pushes tests, procedures, medicines, and specialization.

One can envision geriatric ERs and ACE units with palliative care teams in which the ill elderly can be cared for compassionately to stabilize them before sending them home with home-care services. Currently hospitals are potentially harmful destinations for older patients that offer no measurable medical benefit in many cases. Medicare both generously reimburses hospital care and encourages hospitalization through its payment system. It does very little to help with home care and other focused medical interventions provided outside an aggressive hospital setting. The cost of hospital care for the elderly is one of the most potent factors draining Medicare of its funding without delivering any value. For that reality to change, Medicare must orchestrate a saner course.

5

Long-Term Care

The Unwitting Geriatric ICU

Too often in these institutions, there is more attention paid to disease than to persons, more scientific curiosity about the machinery of the body than consideration of the human values that make life worthwhile.

NORTIN HADLER, *Rethinking Aging*

Long-term care is the soul of geriatrics. It is in long-term care facilities that we care for the frailest of the elderly. We see them in their homes at all hours of the day, we joke with them, sit with them, and often hold their hands during times of extreme emotions. Many of them have dementia, and as they drift away from reality we become an integral part of their new lives, and those of their loved ones. I take care of people in many assisted-living and nursing facilities. Some are small homes managed by good-natured owners and nursing aides, others are large national chains or independent facilities with administrators, nurses, and aides who are equally devoted to their residents. We all work as a team, and all of us enjoy immersing ourselves in the lives of those for whom we care. It is a huge responsibility, and one that none of us takes lightly. Nothing gives us more joy than having our patients smile when we walk by, or talk to us about their past lives, or walk with us serenely on the way to breakfast. I have become close to all the people in my facilities—social workers, aides, nurses, therapists, administrators, patients, families, and so many others. Caring for the residents of long-term care is a passion that many of us in geriatrics share.

There are many types of long-term care. Assisted-living facilities typically house those who can perform some tasks on their own, although increasingly they are being occupied by people with significant mental and physical limitations. Many larger homes have separate dementia units, where residents with more severe dementia live in various arrangements. The cost of assisted-living facilities varies, though typically they are less expensive than nursing homes. They are also less regulated than nursing homes, cannot care for skilled residents, as we will discuss, and are typically self-pay, rarely admitting more than a few residents for whom Medicaid pays all the bills. Nursing homes typically are much larger. Some have hundreds of beds, ventilation units, and even dialysis on the premises. Nursing homes are highly regulated and they hire an expansive staff to care for residents and comply with regulations. The typical resident of a nursing home is more impaired, usually with severe dementia, and requiring a significant amount of custodial care. When residents exhaust their funds, Medicaid may pay for their stay, although many nursing homes actually lose money on their Medicaid residents. Where they earn more money is in Medicare payment, something that creates yet another layer of regulation. Any Medicare patient who stays three nights in a hospital who then has a skilled need (nursing care or physical therapy) can qualify for up to one hundred days of services within a nursing home paid by Medicare. Often nursing homes need a significant number of skilled Medicare residents to offset the cost of their unskilled Medicaid residents.

If there are any places on this earth where older patients should be treated with a minimalistic approach, where adverse outcomes should be expected and ameliorated palliatively without looking for cause or ascribing blame, where trips to the hospital should be avoided at all costs, where medicines and tests should be shunned, and where comfort and dignity should be the only goals, it is at long-term care facilities. And yet it is at such facilities that I have seen aggressive care reach its zenith. We will primarily be discussing nursing homes in this chapter, since assisted-living facilities are less burdened by state regulations and Medicare rules, but assisted-living facilities are not unfettered by the shackles placed on all long-term care facilities, and many of them too are forced to maintain an aggressive stance.

Everything we know about geriatrics tells us that number chasing, overly thorough testing and treatment, and hospitalization in this population is counterproductive, often leading to more harm than good. And yet facility patients are flooded by thorough care incessantly, much more than they would be if they lived at home. Although hardly alone in its culpability, Medicare plays a large role in pushing long-term-care patients on a path of aggression. The three-day hospital rule establishes a kind of class system within the nursing-home world, whereby those patients who have had their tickets punched in the hospital are more profitable to a nursing home than those who have not. In all facilities it is far less expensive for facility and patient alike to hospitalize very ill non-skilled residents, also due to Medicare's payment model, while new rules discourage hospitalizing skilled residents at least for the initial month of their stay.

Long-term-care facilities are also burdened by extensive regulations that reward "thorough" care and hospitalization and rebuke a more palliative approach. This, more than even Medicare's rules, firmly roots aggressive treatment in the culture of long-term care. As with Medicare's quality indicators, discussed in chapter 1, the regulatory environment relies on numbers and scales to assess quality. Whether from state or federal regulations or Medicare's own regulatory assessment tools, these quality indicators span hundreds of pages and are difficult for even the most seasoned administrators to fully comprehend. But the upshot of their message is that poor outcomes are not tolerated, that every facet of an elderly resident's health must be constantly monitored and maintained in the "normal" range, and that failure to comply with the regulations can lead to very damaging consequences. In my experience, compliance with regulatory demands uses up more of frontline staff members' time than patient care does; charting has become the primary activity on a nursing-home floor. Even more significantly, all of us who care for the residents have to worry as much about numbers and regulatory deficiencies as we do the health and well-being of our patients.

The modus operandi of long-term care is specialization. Although specialist doctors do not typically meander the halls of long-term care facilities, and the majority of patients there are treated by geriatric primary-care doctors and nurse practitioners who are well versed in palliative care, long-term-care culture is one of myopic intensity, where a holistic outlook dissolves amid a thorough assault on every ailment, numerical deviation, and complaint exhibited by the frail elderly residents and those who care for them. Palliative care exists only when patients are deemed to be on the verge of death and enrolled in hospice. As is common in specialized environments, patients are carved up into diagnoses and conditions, each one viewed independently from the others, and each one treated aggressively. Tests and procedures are common within the walls of long-term care, with lab and X-ray technicians making frequent trips there, medications tossed at patients for every numerical blip or complaint, and hospitalization natural consequence of medical problems that become difficult to control. Short of the hospital itself, long-term-care facilities are the most specialized settings I have practiced in.

Of course, from everything we have discussed in this book, one has to wonder why the specialized model of care has taken root in long-term care, when its frail elderly inhabitants are most potentially harmed by narrowly focused aggressive care, and when palliation would seem to be most humane and effective. For instance, is it truly necessary to check blood pressures and sugars, often several times a day, and to assure that those pressures fall within a preordained range lest the nurses become alarmed and demand immediate intense treatment? What evidence exists that such thorough numerical monitoring actually benefits the frail elderly and that its treatment helps quality of life or even longevity? And if an older patient passes out, appears more tired, presents with stroke-like symptoms, or becomes more confused, what evidence exists that exposing such elderly patients to copious testing and hospitalization, where precise causes of each problem are ascertained by probing their aged bodies, will improve outcome and quality? Yet that is precisely what happens regularly in long-term care. And Medicare pays for it all. While some Medicare reform is targeting the excessive hospitalization to which long-term-care residents are subjected, nothing has been suggested to alter the specialized model of care within such facilities and to change the rules and financial realities that promote such aggressive care.

Ironically, those who manage the long-term-care facilities in which I work, from owners to administrators, from nurses to aides, from social workers to nurse practitioners and doctors, do not endorse the aggressive cloud under which we have been asked to work. Some of the most progressive, creative, and humane geriatric thinkers I have ever encountered are the owners and directors of long-term-care facilities, one of whom helped me start my practice and who has guided me along the way, inspiring me with his conception of an ideal geriatric universe that he has tried so hard to implement against a tide of resistance. We are all victims of a system that has morphed into something other than what it was designed to be.

Regulation

There is always a healthy debate in this country about how much regulation is too much. In the nursing-home world, that answer is obvious to many of us who practice geriatrics: the *quantity* of regulations in nursing homes, and to a lesser extent assisted-living facilities, is excessive, and the *quality* of such regulation is both poor and counterproductive. Nursing homes are some of the most highly regulated institutions in the country.[1] In fact, regulations frequently trump the good patient care that nursing homes are trying to promote. Facilities spend excessive money and resources to make sure they are in compliance with the hundreds of regulations, leaving less money and fewer resources to spend on their residents' actual care, including hiring more aides and ensuring staff retention.

What are the regulations? Before my first state survey as a medical director I saw the facility director and several nurses walking around with a tape measure to determine if the spacing of items on the wall was within the guidelines. Even though the nursing home was contending with its usual array of significant clinical problems among its residents, the surveyors that year were focusing on measurements, and thus the facility had to devote more resources to that meaningless issue.

Every fall; every piece of tissue-paper skin that tears in a ninety-year-old; every resident who requires a sedative to keep him from screaming all night; every piece of paper that is not signed in the right place at the right time; every chart sitting on the wrong part of a desk; not enough pain medicine; too much pain medicine; constipation from pain medicine; every mistake that occurs, however inadvertent and minor; every complaint by an angry family member—all of these cause consternation among nursing-home administrators because any one of them can lead to a regulatory error, which can trigger a large fine, which can downgrade a facility in its rating, and which can precipitate financial hurt. I am contacted throughout the day and night by many facilities, often with minor issues like a weight change, a slightly elevated blood pressure, a normal lab result, or a fall. I am asked to respond immediately with a plan of correction that can be documented and charted, all in the name of regulatory compliance.

I conducted an exhaustive literature search to see whether any evidence exists tying nursing-home regulation to quality. Unfortunately, the answer to that query is predicated on how "quality" is defined. Since regulations define quality by numbers—how many falls, how many psychiatric medicines people are on, how many urine infections, how many forms are not signed—then clearly by that definition quality is improved with the regulations. It is a self-fulfilling conclusion, and one that seems to have hampered the true objectivity of any study that assesses the quality of care in long-term-care facilities. But do those numbers truly represent quality? To me, more significant measures of patient quality—happiness, social interaction, energy, fewer outbursts by residents, fewer trips to the hospital, less pain—are not genuinely addressed. Several studies that do take a broader view of geriatric care note a disappointing relationship between quality of care and the regulatory environment.[2] Using the commonsense measures we have addressed in this book as indicators of quality geriatric care, I conclude that regulation not only does not contribute to better care, it actually detracts from it.

There is a second layer of regulation that exhausts resources within a nursing home. To be paid by Medicare for skilled services, and to achieve the highest payment that Medicare allows, facilities must comply with a complex set of rules, many of which also require copious documentation of time, numbers, scales, and grades. As with state regulatory rules, the failure of a nursing home to comply with Medicare rules can be financially perilous. Thus homes hire a squadron of staff to help as much with regulation compliance as with patient care. Any visit to the nursing station at a nursing home or even assisted-living facility will typically find doctors and nurses sitting in front of computers charting and compiling data more than actively caring for our patients. While we enjoy each other's company as we sit for hours mindlessly entering information into preset templates on our computers, we would rather be sitting with our patients or having more time to talk to families. Regulations, however, make that impossible.

Number Obsession

Numbers in particular are placed under a microscope in facilities. They are easy to measure, and thus easy to regulate, even if they typically lack clinical significance. Today I was told that an assisted-living patient was on the regulatory radar because, according to a county social worker who was scrutinizing the facility, his blood pressure was too high and he should have a diagnosis of hypertension and be on blood pressure medicine. In my opinion the pressure was perfectly fine and we had no reason to treat it, let alone even check it. What the regulator was requesting would have been detrimental to the patient, for reasons we have already discussed. The social worker went ever further, arguing that since the patient had a diagnosis of high cholesterol on her problem list, we were being negligent in not having her on statin drugs and checking her cholesterol labs tests periodically. We satisfied the regulator by removing both diagnoses from the problem list and by my writing a note explaining that the pressure and cholesterol were normal for her age and medical condition.

I have many constructive debates with nurses about numbers. Often I am hounded by various voices in a facility because I refuse to treat what they consider high sugars and high blood pressure. I beg the nurses to stop checking blood pressure so often and I try hard to prevent any but the most essential sugar checks. I cite studies, which we have discussed in this book, demonstrating that aggressive treatment of hypertension and diabetes in frail elderly residents of long-term-care facilities leads to worse functional outcomes, but those facts do not deflect the reality of long-term-care regulations, even though the nurses and I are almost always in agreement. When a regulator spots "untreated" high blood pressure or diabetes, or vital signs and labs tests that are not being ordered in sufficient quantity, then she may fault a facility and instigate a painful and potentially expensive citation process. When regulators play doctor and set the rules, nurses really have no choice but to comply.

blood pressure increased every day, and she became more confused and agitated. A speech therapist was consulted, who similarly questioned her safety. That caused nurses to march into her room day and night looking worried and rolling beeping blood-pressure machines at their sides. They called me and her son with panic, telling us that she was choking, that she was coughing, reading her blood pressures and weights, and requesting medicines, X-rays, even hospitalization. Her son became more anxious.

"Maybe we need to get her to a hospital," he asked me one day. "Maybe they're right."

"Just hold the course," I told him. "Nothing has changed. She is fine."

Then came the director of nursing and social workers, asking her if she wanted a feeding tube, telling her that she may die without it. Her anxiety level increased even further. Then the medical director intervened. A doctor himself, whose role in long-term care was to ensure that all doctors complied with state and facility regulations and that facility physicians adhered to quality geriatric care (two goals that often are contradictory), he directly inserted himself into the situation. He talked to the patient and son and told them that she may well die if she did not get a tube put in her stomach to feed her immediately, that waiting for the surgery could be fatal, and that he could arrange for the tube to be put in. Certainly he was acting at the request of the administrators, who feared reprisals from regulators, and who were uncomfortable with a woman who could have an adverse outcome. Of course, the son became frantic, and the level of anxiety literally exploded.

I told the son not to worry. I came in early the next morning and wrote a two-page note in the chart explaining that the medical director was completely out of line to insert himself in a situation he did not understand, that the nurses and administrators needed to back off, and that the patient was doing fine by every objective criterion we had, including weight (which had not dropped since admission) and blood work. My words were sharp, and I was reprimanded by the medical director, and in fact was almost fired for my actions. Two weeks later the woman had her surgery, went home with twenty-four-hour care rather than returning to the nursing home, and lived very well (out of hospitals and subsequent nursing homes) for the rest of her life, which spanned many years.

Falls: The Benefits of Frontline Staff

Many residents move to long-term care because they fall, and thus it is not a surprise that they are still falling after they arrive. Many have dementia and try to get up even though they should not. They need to go to the bathroom and will not or cannot wait. Sometimes their blood pressure is too low, they are on too many medicines, or they are on medicines known to cause falls.[4] Having more nursing aides around, and having residents in activities that are monitored, can mitigate the chance of falling. But there are never enough aides to help everyone, and regulatory law prevents restraining residents. Even when medicines are used to calm them, that only increases their rates of falls. And because falls trigger regulatory alarms, facilities have to be very attentive to them. Fall-prevention programs can help,[5] but their implementation requires money and trained personnel, something lacking in facilities that have to devote so many resources to nonclinical activities, such as regulatory and Medicare compliance.

I was amazed to learn one day at a nursing home that its corporate administration was looking into the reason that so many nursing-home residents were falling by spending $500,000 to hire a consultant to ascertain the cause of falls. I was floored. I remember sitting around with some of the nursing aides one morning talking about it.

"They fall," one of them said, "because they all have to go to the bathroom at the same time, and we can't all be there at that time for every one of them." She had been at the nursing home for a long time, one of the few aides who actually stayed for more than a year. "I know I have to see Mrs. S. right away when she gets up, then hurry to Mr. W., then I told Mrs. L. to be patient, and I know she usually won't try to get up until I get there while the other two will, but sometimes she just does anyway."

"If they took that money they're paying that consultant and just hired some more aides," another one said, "then the problem would be solved tomorrow."

"If they took some of that money and paid us just a little more, then we would stick around and that would solve the problem too," another chimed in.

Yes, the nursing aides solved the whole problem in a matter of minutes. Pay nurses and aides enough to induce them to remain loyal so that they stay, thereby ensuring that they know their patients and that their patients/

families know them. Make sure there are enough nurses and aides so that they can help people when help is needed and can get a break once in a while, because taking care of an old nursing-home-resident who slaps you and who greets you with a diaper full of excrement is not the most pleasant way to spend a day, and there are always a few of those in every nursing home with whom aides have to contend. And treat the nurses and aides with dignity and respect. Too often aides are blamed when problems occur, they are fired, they are reprimanded, and the system chews them up like they are just pegs in some grand board game.

The cost of having more and happier frontline staff is minimal compared to what some facilities pay their executives and consultants to try to solve weighty issues such as fall prevention, and that cost translates into a better facility. When average annual turnover of nursing aides is above 85 percent, quality will clearly decline.[6] There is nothing more revealing than the reaction of patients and families when they lose their trusted aide. In my experience patients demonstrate sadness, consternation, fear, and usually a worsening of behavior. Regulators do not measure that level of quality, but we see it every day.

Interestingly, while good aides clearly help improve a facility and resident/family satisfaction, it does not necessarily lead to a better regulatory outcome. One study I read suggested that increasing the number of nursing aides in a facility does not lead to fewer deficiencies on a state survey,[7] likely because the survey process is measuring parameters that do not reflect the quality that aides deliver. Aides can engage with residents in interesting and personalized activities, walk with them, sing and laugh with them, make them feel happy and autonomous, and be more attuned to their needs, but there may be no appreciable improvement in most survey quality indicators. In fact, when facilities permit residents to have more freedom, where they are not watched like hawks and they are involved in creative dementia programs, falls may increase, especially when there are not enough aides to personally watch every high-risk resident all the time.

Medicines and Regulatory Schizophrenia

Pharmaceutical regulations are also very vexing and cost facilities money and time to ensure compliance. These regulations are often contradictory, demanding more lab tests, number measurements, and medicines, even as they chastise polypharmacy. Patients are not permitted to be in pain, and yet the regulations required to maintain patients on pain medicines are arduous and time-consuming for everyone in the facilities. Similarly, facilities would like to ensure that very confused, agitated, and even delusional residents are relatively calm, do not bother other residents, do not fall, and shower and eat regularly, but facilities are often denied the tools to make that happen. Nurses and nursing aides are put in a horrible position as some residents lash out at them or start to run off, and it requires half of a floor of staff to try to redirect them without using restraints or coercion, which the regulations forbid. They also do not typically have enough time to provide the personal attention to calm and redirect confused residents. So we treat them with medicines, most of which are not indicated for dementia, carry a black-box warning, and lead to sedation and falls. Regulations frown on such medicines, while at the same time frowning on what would happen should those medicines not be given. It's damned if you do and damned if you don't in the medical universe of long-term care.

Every medicine carries a potential risk, and every medicine can lead to regulatory issues if specified rules about its use are not followed. Some medicines require lab surveillance, some require attempts at stopping them periodically, some need special forms that doctors must complete frequently, while others are felt to be inappropriate for the elderly and require us to justify their use. Therefore facilities have to employ specific long-term-care pharmacies to dispense their medicines and provide a consultant pharmacist. The pharmacist reviews charts regularly and instructs facilities on how to follow the regulatory rules. While a little input from a pharmacist is always invited, and the pharmacists with whom I work are wonderful people who educate us and help us remain compliant, these guidelines, which flow to us frequently in the form of reports we have to address, are born of regulatory needs, not of any true adherence to quality geriatric care. They also cost patients more money, since medicine prices are escalated to cover the regulatory expense, and they cost the facility both time and money. They also lead to excessive number obsession, test ordering, and second-guessing.

Facilities are also forbidden from dispensing over-the-counter medicines without a doctor's order. If my knee hurts I can take a Tylenol, and if my nose runs I can take a Claritin. But long-term-care residents require doctor orders for everything, even a vitamin. If we add a bunch of basic over-the-counter medicines to the patient's list that can be dispensed as needed, that also causes consternation since facilities are judged too on how long their average resident's medicine list is. They must remain on four blood-pressure medicines and a statin because we of course need to keep the numbers looking good, but God forbid we add a few medicines for constipation, pain, heartburn, or gas that they can get when they ask. Comfort takes a back seat to regulatory requirements and number fixing.

The Survey: Regulation's Annual Alamo

In some distant past life I am sure that facility regulations were developed to prevent gross negligence and excess. Some facilities were certainly mistreating residents and scamming the system. But these days, the vast majority of the facilities are doing their best to take care of a very sick patient population in a responsible and dignified way. I have never been to a facility that deserved anything but a high passing grade on a state survey. While regulators can assess facilities at any time, and people are monitoring falls and dozens of other numbers regularly, the big survey occurs only once a year (and less frequently in assisted-living facilities). Survey day is never announced, but facilities are given a window of several months in which a squadron of regulators could potentially arrive, and there is always talk among the many facilities in a community speculating when the regulators may be nearby. Anxiety grips facilities as soon as there's a hint that the regulatory team may be close. Nurses, social workers, and administrators spend long days and often some nights digging through charts, putting everything in its place, making sure that every bad outcome is accounted for and every paper is signed.

On survey day the entire facility essentially bows down to the all-powerful regulators, holding its collective breath as a small squadron enters the building, skewers the charts, talks to people, digs into every nook and cranny of the floor, and then starts handing out deficiencies. On our last survey, the regulators determined that some pages in a chart were not signed. A deficiency was allocated. The facility then spent the next few months not only fixing that problem, but developing a new system to ensure that the problem would not occur again, and then proving to the regulators that the new system (a binder in which unsigned pages were kept for every doctor) was being used by sending them a plan of correction. It was a huge waste of money and time for nothing! And that was a good survey!

Last summer I spent days grappling with a survey result that cited us because our office note indicated that a patient was on an over-the-counter medicine but the facility chart did not have that medicine listed. This required hours of phone time, written letters, and meetings before it was resolved, although a deficiency was still handed to the facility. Recently I witnessed a survey team citing a facility because a two-hundred-pound woman fell on a nursing aide as the aide was trying desperately to transfer her out of the bed; the facility fired the aide, likely so that blame could be deflected from it to her. On one occasion a daughter complained that her mom fell too many times. In reality, despite the aide's best efforts, the mom would try to get up as soon as the aide left the room. The regulators paid a visit. That aide was fired. On another occasion a facility received a survey deficiency because an aide was yelling loudly at a resident with dementia, even though the resident in question was deaf and refused to wear her hearing aids.

As soon as an annual survey is complete, the facility is already preparing for the next one. Facilities are given one to five stars based primarily on survey results. People like to put their loved ones in five-star facilities. So the facility administrator will do everything in his or her power to get to four or five stars. In addition to causing star reduction, survey deficiencies incur fines, some of which are very large. Deficiencies also mandate facilities engage in a process that proceeds for several months after the survey, whereby they have to write a comprehensive evaluation of why they were deficient and what plan of correction they intend to implement to ensure it does not happen again. I remember sitting in monthly quality-assurance meetings as the charge nurse had to read her plan of correction month after month, explaining what was being done to fix the cited problem: having a cookie-warming machine to give residents cookies in a patient-care area, something the survey thought could be dangerous. Such deficiencies squander valuable time for nurses and aides who would rather concentrate on patient needs and talk about creative ways to care for their residents instead of having to focus on the placement of unplugged cookie-warming machines.

A few months ago I was giving a talk to nurses and aides about how to address residents with dementia who refuse care, are agitated, and are unable to be redirected. We discussed the need to avoid confronting such residents when they resist certain aspects of care and not to stress them by arguing with them. We talked about psychiatric medicines, their side effects, and how regulations impact their use. And we talked about checking certain labs and tests and urines when residents do become more confused. One aide who had been there for a while told us how she dealt with one of the most agitated residents on the floor. The resident would not eat, and would not shower; she swung at people who tried to direct her. So the aide, who knew the resident and family well, learned something about her life. Before every shower day she told the resident that it was prom night, and that her prom date would be here soon. The resident lit up with glee, and cheerfully took a shower and dressed herself. Then she ate. This happened day after day. She did not need medicines, labs, tests, probes, blood-pressure cuffs, consultants, or hospital admission to solve a difficult problem. Rather, because she knew the resident well, because she asked the right questions, and because she cared, the underpaid nursing aide employed compassion and common sense to make someone happy in her last months or years on this earth. It is very likely that the survey process would frown on her approach; after all, she did lie to the resident almost every day. But what the survey fails to grasp is that the best form of medicine is not a series of numbers and deficiencies that can be measured and charted, but something much more ephemeral. It is good geriatric care. It is love. And that comes often at less expense.

Expectations Gone Wild

In the nursing-home environment, although most of my patients and their children truly value comfort and dignity as the primary goals of care, many others are imbued with a belief that number chasing and aggressive treatment are both appropriate and beneficial. I remember taking one of my older patients off a statin cholesterol drug when she developed a severe bronchitis and had trouble walking. This was a patient who requested frequent labs tests and medicines, and nothing I could say would dissuade her from the perception that more is better. But now, in the midst of her lung infection, I believed that the statin was actually causing her harm, so I persuaded her to stop it.

"That medicine could make you hurt more," I told her. "I'm going to remove it."

She acceded but was very sick, and I am not sure she fully comprehended the ramifications of my words.

Months later, having forgotten our conversation, a nurse told her that her statin was gone from her medicine list. She screamed at me, telling me that I was trying to kill her, that I didn't have any sense or knowledge, accusing me of not giving old people good care. I tried to explain that we could start it again, that being off a cholesterol medicine for a few months would cause no harm, and that at the time she benefited from its discontinuation. But she wanted none of my rationalizations; after all, someone had put her on that pill to save her life, and now I had callously removed it. She immediately fired me and found a new doctor, one who was more thorough. I remember sitting at the nursing station a few weeks later, when she rolled in with her electric wheelchair. Pointing at me, but talking to the nurse, she said, "Does that nincompoop still work here?"

Several times a year I publish a newsletter in my practice discussing updated issues in geriatric care. This year I wrote my back-page article on excessive care in the nursing home. Discussing recent studies and citing my own experience, I concluded that many people in long-term care are better served through a palliative approach that does not emphasize fixing numbers and sending people to the hospital.

Soon enough I heard concerns voiced about my article. One of my patients asked another doctor if I was trying to kill people who got old, like Dr. Kevorkian. Another patient of mine brought over a written statement to me declaring that she wanted everything done for her should she get sick, so fearful was she that I would pull the plug the moment illness struck her. To these and other patients, the idea that palliation could actually be beneficial flies in the face of what they believe is good care. My audacity in arguing for a minimalistic approach was interpreted as cruel and unfeeling.

The idea of long-term care as being a "rest home" or "convalescent home" has morphed over the decades. Now there can be no rest when monitors, needles, X-rays, and medicines are thrust at long-term-care residents steadily. "Rest home" is the very antithesis of what these places have become.

Mrs. H. learned that lesson quickly. Her husband Mr. H.'s dementia progressed slowly. Mrs. H. kept him busy playing tennis, engaged with friends, and reading history books. But as his disease advanced, she watched his brilliant and energetic mind wilt away, and she saw her own vibrant life torn apart by his accelerating confusion and disability. During the early stages of his disease Mrs. H., who attended most of his appointments, made sure her husband spent at least part of every visit with me alone. He always joked that the most annoying part of his disease was that the uneducated ladies with whom he ate dinner could talk and reason better than he could, even though they talked out of their asses. One day he told me point blank that if his Alzheimer's advanced to the point that his wife needed to care for him at the expense of her own life, or that he could not hold his own in a conversation, he intended to take out one of his guns and blow out his brains. His visage exuded absolute determination.

When I relayed his sentiments to his wife, she smiled and shrugged her shoulders. "Who can blame him?" she said to me.

Like so many spouses of my dementia patients, Mrs. H. made a heroic stand against her husband's disease. She read about dementia, talked to me regularly about how to handle certain behavioral problems he exhibited, and kept her husband busy, always respecting his dignity. But unlike so many spouses, Mrs. H. knew when to say when. She did not chase elusive cures or flood him with feckless medicines. When their existence was transformed into a perpetual day-care center, when he embarrassed himself by soiling his pants in public or babbling nonsensically during conversations, Mrs. H. reluctantly moved the proud but bewildered man into a nursing home. She had cared for him for almost a decade at home, and now her husband barely could string together a meaningful sentence. He had moved well beyond the ability to kill himself or even generate such a complex thought. Mrs. H. asked me to stop all his medicines and treat him for nothing but pain. She wanted to give him peace.

The nurses questioned her harsh stance; Mr. H. looked good, seemed happy, and was very engaging. But she knew he did not want to live this way. When he stopped eating, she told me that was his choice, and she wanted no intervention. When he developed pneumonia, she told me to keep him comfortable, not to give him antibiotics. People in the nursing home questioned her position. From nurses to administrators, the nursing home pounced on her for neglecting her husband.

"They keep telling me I am doing the wrong thing," she told me, refer-ring to the nursing-home staff and administrators. "They tell me that I am letting him die."

We talked about it. She felt horribly guilty. Often in my experience, even when a patient's family member reaches a decision to allow nature take its course, she is pushed hard to be more aggressive not only by the facility, but also by other family and friends. Mrs. H. was a strong woman who held her own ground. She knew what was best for her husband, and when he did die, he did so peacefully. Dementia is a tragic disease. Mrs. H. had lost her husband years earlier, but she could not mourn him. She stood by helplessly as her husband's illness ripped out his soul and left an empty hide in his place. This is the last thing he would have wanted. Finally, knowing that their love needed a release, she became a hero and let her husband go. But that approach did not sit well in the do-everything world of long-term care. In fact, to many it seemed cruel, as I heard in the echoes of the staff's chatter after his death, none of which was complimentary to Mrs. H.

I recall another patient with severe dementia, Mrs. L., whose husband cared for her as best he could. Both were lovely people. But when a sudden illness overcame and weakened her, he sent her to the nursing home. She did not recover. He made the conscious decision to treat her only for pain and discomfort, eschewing more aggressive care. His daughters were not happy with the decision. They talked to the nurses and learned that their mom had stopped eating and refused to walk. The nurses and staff out-lined many steps that could be taken: blood tests, urine tests, chest X-rays, hospitalization. They told the daughters that their father refused all such care. One of the daughters talked to me and, with the permission of Mrs. L.'s husband, who was also my patient, I told them that I agreed with his decisions, as both he and his wife had told me that they did not want any extraordinary care once they had reached the end of life.

"How do you know she is at the end of life?" the daughter asked me. "How does he know? Why not give her a chance?"

I tried to explain to her that even if we found something wrong and fixed it, there was a slim chance that her deteriorating body could be re-vived. We might delay her death, but it would not be for long. When an older person with dementia turns off, when she stops eating and interact-ing, we can mine for problems and repair them, one after another, but only at the cost of causing her pain and triggering even more problems, and never with the likelihood of inducing any real healing. She listened, but I do not think she accepted my words. The nurses told her that there were other options to explore. Her friends implored her to do more. How could her dad let Mom die without a fight?

So she fought her dad, making him more miserable. He was very firm in his conviction, repeating to me and to his daughters that his wife had insisted she not be treated with anything more than comfort should she become incapacitated. He had documents to prove it, which was good because otherwise his stand would have been more difficult. So his daughter stopped talking to him. She also stopped talking to her sister, who decided to support her dad. When my patient finally died several weeks later, it took many months before the once close family came back together.

I have seen countless families torn apart by such wrenching decisions. Many families of long-term-care residents find it difficult to abandon hope, which is how they perceive the relinquishing of an aggressive mentality, even if their loved one had previously told them to act otherwise. There is always more that can be done, more tests and treatments, even a hospital stay, that can perhaps reverse the slide that aging has instigated. They have heard stories about other people in similar circumstances who, when at death's door, were treated and cured. Society bombards them with tales of hope as long as they never abandon their fight. The nursing-home environment only reinforces that mentality and eggs them on.

Pushed to the Brink

It is almost twilight-zone-like for a geriatric doctor to watch all the medical attention being showered on the frailest residents of long-term care who are trying so hard to just be comfortable while probes and needles are being shoved into them or the ambulance squad is throwing them on a gurney for a long and bumpy ride to the hospital. And that level of intensity pushes everyone—families, nurses, doctors, patients—into a state of mind whereby anxiety and high expectations completely obscure common sense and geriatric reality.

Because of regulatory rules, families are often bombarded by concerns about their loved ones from nurses and staff, especially if their family member has become more ill, and these families then start to worry. Sometimes they watch mom decline and wonder why, thinking there is more that could and should be done, that no one should ever die or decline without more of an effort, perhaps even a stay in the hospital. The long-term-care environment feeds their angst. Once panic starts to overtake reason, once the fable of hope supplants the reality of aging, then there is no turning back. As a doctor in those situations I am often barraged by emails and calls, from nurses, from families, even from other physicians. They crescendo in intensity, day and night, dramatizing the extent of the resident's medical collapse, requesting that more be done, often pushing for hospitalization. In my more idealistic youth I would try to convince them that staying put was the best approach, and sometimes I would come into the facility to try to be more persuasive. That approach could delay the inevitable for hours, maybe a day, but I soon learned that once the fear and panic take over, they will never be stopped. Now I typically just give up and send them off to the hospital.

Just yesterday a ninety-three-year-old woman presented at the office with what seemed to be a small stroke, and I discussed the options of both hospitalization and nonskilled-nursing-home placement with her and her son. She adamantly opposed the hospital, but it took some convincing to persuade her son, who had heard that a patient must be sent to the hospital without pause if they had signs of stroke. Calling 911 would have been easy and my day would have been done. Instead we set up a CT scan that evening and arranged an admission to a long-term-care facility, something that took hours of time, and something for which the family would have to pay. The next day a physical therapist told the son that not going to the hospital was a poor decision. He started to see a decline in his mom, something reinforced reluctantly by nursing. Vital signs were abnormal. She could not swallow correctly. She likely became more nervous as everyone around her worried. A wave of anxiety consumed the son and the entire floor. Why wasn't she sent to the hospital? Were we just going to let her die? Somehow, as often happens, the hospital took on a magical power, as though when a ninety-three-year-old stroke victim rolls through its doors her ailments will be expunged miraculously. All our time and effort trying to treat this very elderly woman in the most palliative and humane way possible, and in total concert with her own wishes, collapsed in a matter of hours. An innuendo of doubt sparked the fire, and then more fuel intensified the flames, because in the world of long-term care there is always an abundance of kindling and little available to extinguish a fire once it starts. She was whisked away to the hospital, and there was nothing we could do. In fact, if she survived three nights there, her ticket would be punched and the entire subacute stay would be financed by Medicare. As a colleague told me, it is senseless trying to stop it; I should have just called 911 when she walked in the door.

With so many people magnifying every medical problem into a crisis, with so many rules and incentives hastening nursing-home residents to the nearest hospital, with so much monitoring being done, with so low a level of tolerance for any clinical deterioration, and with so many families who start having unrealistic expectations, no wonder thorough care becomes the norm. No wonder ambulances and X-ray machines and lab technicians make incessant visits to the nursing home. No wonder the level of anxiety and anger is always high, reflecting a shared frustration. And no wonder the cost of geriatric care, both financially and personally, is so much steeper than anywhere else in the medical community.

What makes the facility atmosphere even worse is family frustration with long-term care. Many families I know who send their loved ones into assisted-living facilities or nursing homes do so reluctantly, often with their loved ones kicking and screaming and blaming them. Clearly when they do make the decision for long-term-care placement, families are driven by necessity; their parents can no longer safely or affordably live at home. Not everyone is so blessed as to have the Taunton Portuguese community I worked in years ago that can keep people like Mrs. A. at home, or the resources to hire round-the-clock help. And families have to pay huge fees to send their loved ones to long-term-care facilities, something that often is very stressful as well. When finally the decision is made, and mom or dad is deposited in a small room with a roommate, most family members are already fried. They are struggling enough with their loved one's decline, and now are even more distraught that their loved one has to live the rest of her life in a small room with no autonomy, in a place many of them vowed never to be.

The anger and angst typically accelerate early in their loved one's stay. They come in to find mom sitting in a pool of urine. They learn she fell twice, that she did not eat her breakfast, that she slapped an aide. They see that a food tray is left by her side untouched and assume that no one attempted to feed her. They see that she sits in a chair staring at the wall much of the day. They witness other confused residents wandering into her room. They start to complain to the nurses, to spend more time there. They have lost so much control that they feel helpless and even guiltier. They start to question every aspect of Mom's care.

All of this is augmented when they receive bills from the facility for hidden fees and exorbitant medication costs. They wonder how they will be able to afford this. Then they get calls requesting more medicines, more tests, hearing that Mom's blood pressure has been too high, that she fell twice more at night trying to go to the bathroom, that she is losing weight and may need supplements, and that the doctor thinks she needs a psychiatrist consult for her confusion and agitation. Some calls come early in the morning, some of the people calling are barely able to be understood and often have a sense of panic in their voice. Social workers ask more about advanced directives and living wills and finances, while nurses continue to barrage them with every clinical change that occurs. Everyone is trying to help them, and most families know that, but the situation becomes difficult to bear. The level of tension rises, and slowly many family members are dragged into the long-term-care zeitgeist where illness is not tolerated, where deterioration needs to be addressed aggressively, where there must be a reason for everything that goes wrong.

Virtually every nurse and social worker with whom I work knows the folly of aggressive care in the frail elderly. It often upsets them to have to be party to the assault. Very often, early in a patient's stay, the staff meets with families and discusses the benefit of palliation. Social workers offer forms that help families move down a path of less aggressive care. But families become confused within the contradictory and intense environment that defines long-term care. They are informed about every adverse outcome, every abnormal numerical deviation, every fall and skipped meal. They are often led to believe that they have to choose between aggressive care and death, especially if the specter of hospice is evoked. Often they reach a point of emotional single-mindedness and believe that, with enough effort, Mom will not have to die, a belief that is reinforced by family and friends and the very ethos of US health-care delivery. They resist the palliative approach and demand even more aggressive surveillance and treatment. I have seen this occur even among the frailest of my patients, and among those who explicitly stated that they did not want to be kept alive.

Sometimes even the most pleasant and intelligent family members become indignant about their loved one's decline, and lose trust in everyone claiming to be trying to help and palliate their mom. And at that juncture, a reluctant staff has to become equally thorough in the patient's care, and the cycle of aggression accentuates to the point of no return.

Nothing makes the system even more dysfunctional than an indignant or frustrated family member. The nurses are frightened to do anything less than everything. Administrators are on edge. And their loved ones who live in the facility become more anxious and thus get more confused; they act out, eat less, and have higher blood pressure. I have seen stable people with dementia placed onto the gurney of an ambulance so many times, not because of their own illness but rather the stress and thorough care that is smothering them. What should be a comfortable haven becomes a hellish plunge into medical excess for the residents there.

Take the case of Mrs. S. Her level of dementia was quite high and thus she lived in the nursing home. She was declining by many parameters. She was more confused, losing weight, having elevations of blood pressure, more shortness of breath, and leg swelling. She screamed out often and was resistant to care, including refusing to eat and not allowing aides to wash or dress her. Her daughters were quite aggressive. In the recent past they had brought her to an army of specialists who flooded her with a ton of medicines, all of which she still took. Now, as per family wishes, we ordered X-rays and blood tests frequently. Several times she was sent to the hospital when she seemed on the verge of death, or when her vital signs destabilized, and there her debility only accentuated and nothing of value was accomplished. No definitive cause of the decline was ascertained by even the most thorough testing. Nurses checked daily weights, checked vital signs many times a day, and tried to feed her and persuade her to swallow supplements. All of this only seemed to make her worse. The daughters visited constantly. They tried to push her to eat, to walk, to feel better. They were worried about their mom, whom they loved dearly.

Finally, after many meetings and conversations with doctors, nurses, and social workers, they decided to put their mom on hospice. They did not want her in a hospital again or to be artificially fed, something reflected in her living will. After much hand-holding and reassurance, the daughters agreed to stop their mom's medicines and to keep her comfortable.

No more blood tests, X-rays, weights, or vital signs were taken. Mrs. S. ate only when and what she wanted.

Within weeks Mrs. S. started to improve. She was brighter, happier, and less confused. She ate much better. Her daughters smiled and laughed with her, instead of fussing over her as they had before, and she clearly enjoyed that. Nurses talked to her and laughed with her, rather than putting on blood pressure cuffs and trying to push food down her throat. She enjoyed that too. She became herself again, talking more, becoming more interactive, and not yelling out.

After a few months of steady improvement, and ultimately the decision by hospice to dismiss Mrs. S. due to the fact she no longer was declining, one of the daughters approached me. "Now that Mom is better," she asked, "shouldn't we put her back on her medicines? I am afraid her blood pressure may get too high, and her cholesterol too." I just had to chuckle. She did not get it. Few people do. The medicines and treatments and stress were killing her, not her alleged problems. And now they wanted to instigate the whole cascade all over again.

The Medicare Trap

As I write this chapter I am grappling with a similar situation, but one that is instigated by Medicare itself. Mrs. R., a pleasant woman from an assisted-living facility who had baseline dementia, suffered a severe stroke that left her paralyzed on her left side, unable to talk, and unable to swallow. The hospital doctor persuaded her daughter to surgically place a feeding tube into her gut with the hope that these bags of liquid nutrition would keep her alive long enough to allow her to recover. The daughter acceded to this, not to prolong her life but rather to buy her some time. She was in the hospital for three days, so she was sent to a nursing rehabilitation unit with a "skilled" status, meaning that Medicare would pay most of the bill as long as she remained skilled.

But Mrs. R.'s condition only deteriorated in the rehabilitation facility. She was stricken with bouts of pneumonia from the liquid nutrition rushing up her esophagus and into her lungs, not an uncommon scenario in tube-fed stroke victims. She developed a painful bedsore on her buttocks from a lack of mobility. Her weakness had given no hint of improving. She could not talk or otherwise express herself. As the weeks progressed, and she became further trapped in a body afflicted with discomfort, we could all see a deep sense of hopelessness overtake her.

Mrs. R.'s daughter is reasonable, and she agrees that the time has come to withdraw care, but there is a catch.

As long as Mrs. R. receives tube feeds, Medicare will pay her nursing-home bill. She is considered "skilled," which is a ticket punch for payment. But if the feeding is stopped, or if Mrs. R. enrolls in hospice, Medicare A will drop Mrs. R., and the $300 daily nursing-home bill falls into her daughter's lap. The daughter came to my office in tears. She wants to pull the tube and set up hospice. But she simply cannot afford it. Medicare will only help her if she acts in a way that she knows is contrary to her mother's wishes and contrary to compassionate care. The system has trapped her.

The "skilled" status that was created by Medicare to enable payment for rehabilitation in a nursing home after a significant illness has itself become a trigger for aggressive care in long-term care. It is far less costly for a long-term-care facility to send a sick patient to the hospital rather than treat them in the facility, even if the medical system (and Medicare) has to pay much, much more to treat people in the hospital. Very sick residents exhaust too many resources, making them time drains for nurses and aides, demanding levels of care that are often far too expensive both for the facility and for families. Sick dementia residents often do not eat, they need IV fluids and medicines, they act out and refuse care, they scream and bite. Facilities are frequently forced to ask families to hire private aides for severely ill residents, or to agree to pay for the IVs and other extra care that Medicare does not cover, something that is not only expensive but can irritate a family who is already paying a lot. Once patients go to the hospital and have their tickets punched for three nights, then the family pays less, and the facility gets paid significantly more. True, society has to pay a lot more to send such a patient to the hospital, and it is often the wrong thing to do for an older patient with dementia, but financial reality trumps common sense. It saves everyone money and relieves nursing homes from stress. To watch an old, frail patient with dementia being put on a gurney and dragged kicking and screaming to a hospital, where he will be exposed to illness and excessive intervention, is painful but understandable given the realities of our reimbursement system.

Take the example of pneumonia and dehydration. I have had nursing-home patients who develop pneumonia, but are stable. They are not eating well, but can manage with a lot of help. Sometimes they require intravenous medicine and fluids, something that most facilities can provide, and typically they do need extra care. In fact, studies show that nursing-home patients with pneumonia treated in their own beds do as well as or better than those sent to the hospital.[8] But Medicare does not pay for extra care in the nursing home or assisted-living facility beyond doctor visits. Facilities would need to devote more nursing and aide time to that one patient, taking it away from all the others. It would have to pay to have people manage intravenous lines, often in patients who pull at the lines and cause bleeding and other complications. The medicines and fluids themselves are very expensive for facility and family alike, a cost not covered by Medicare. Rather than suffer all of that, facilities send such patients to the hospital. The benefits for facility and family are immediately apparent. In the hospital Medicare pays for everything. The facility has one fewer sick person to deal with. The family has fewer bills to pay. And if the patient can stay in the hospital three nights and is skilled, suddenly all those expensive medicines and treatments are paid for and the patient returns to the facility with a punched ticket, saving both the facility and the family even more money. Medicare makes everyone a winner with aggressive care!

Forced into the Hospital

Well, there are two losers. One is the taxpaying public who now must foot large Medicare bills to pay for unnecessary and costly hospitalizations. The second is the patient himself, since he will now be exposed to the dangerous hospital. I have seen so many nursing-home residents return from hospitals sicker, more confused, more frail, and having more ailments (resistant infections, bedsores, increased weakness, hospital-acquired diarrhea, to name a few) than when they left. It is clearly safer for them to stay in the nursing home and be treated there, be treated by people who know them, and be kept away from tests, restraints, medical mistakes, inactivity, and bugs that are common in the hospital setting.

We have already discussed how dangerous hospitals can be for elderly patients. The frail elderly who inhabit nursing homes, especially those with dementia, fare even worse. A 2011 *New England Journal of Medicine* study concluded that transitions of nursing-home patients to hospitals are both burdensome "and of limited clinical value." Patients have an increased risk of feeding-tube placement, confusion, inadequate attention to their needs, poor communication, and development of large skin ulcers. Citing the financial pressures that push facilities to send their dementia residents to hospitals despite the risks, the study concludes: "Transitions among patients with advanced dementia are often avoidable because common complications in such patients can be treated with equal efficacy in the nursing home."[9] Medical errors are also common in the transition between nursing home and hospital, causing even more trauma to the vulnerable patient.[10] As we have shown already, with hospitalization dementia and functional status worsen, infections increase, and overall condition can decline among the elderly.

Lawyers

The other catalyst to aggressive treatment that we have already discussed is legal reality. We have all seen commercials on TV with shady lawyers asking if you or a loved one has suffered from nursing-home neglect. The very concept that a nursing home can be sued if a resident suffers a bad outcome is something that most of us have witnessed far too often to simply dismiss. Having felt the sting of a bogus lawsuit personally, I am particularly empathetic to facilities that practice defensive medicine. Why should nursing-home administrators keep potential liabilities in their facility, where adverse outcomes are likely, when they can ship them to hospitals and thus deflect the lawyer's spear? It is always legally prudent to be aggressive, to overtreat and overtest, and to ultimately dump sick people in the hospital.

The financial cost of nursing-home lawsuits is substantial. Concludes one study: "Litigation diverts resources from resident care" due to its excessive cost.[11] Long-term-care facilities that try to improve their atmosphere to enhance resident quality, such as by providing a more homelike environment for dementia residents, are susceptible to liability,[12] likely because they do not follow standard procedures and are not as aggressive with traditional medical care. But such creative approaches to dementia care also afford patients more freedom. Their level of comfort and dignity is much improved, by my observations, and they are less likely to be combative, though from a legal standpoint such patients are facility liabilities.

The Consequences of Thorough

Many of us who work in long-term care innately comprehend the futility of sending our oldest and frailest patients down the road of thorough. We often talk about it with each other, commiserating about our frustration with a system that encourages us to do too much. I have worked with the most wonderful nurses, aides, and social workers, who are underpaid and undervalued given all that they know and do. Every nurse and social worker with whom I have been associated has entered their field for the most noble of reasons, always with the objective to help patients and families. That they have to confront vulnerable families with hard decisions about life and death, with regulations and requirements, with an absurd financial reality, and with mounds of frustrating paperwork is a problem not of their own making. That they have to call families with every adverse outcome and offer hospitalization and aggressive treatment as an option is not something that most nurses desire. Given that the default setting of every long-term-care institution is glued to thorough care, with hospitalization assumed as the best approach for patients who fall too far out of the acceptable norms, we have a hard time nudging patients and families toward a more palliative approach. It requires too much sweat and counterintuitive persuasion and paperwork; it requires families to make too many difficult decisions all at once. It is far easier for everyone just to go with the default.

I conducted an unofficial survey of how many of my long-term-care residents were sent to the hospital during the six weeks that it took to write this chapter. Understand that I do everything I can to avoid hospitalization, that I have a financial incentive to keep them out of the hospital and to see them more frequently in their facility when they are ill, that I have nurse practitioners seeing my patients regularly in facilities in an effort to avert hospitalization, and that I am only one doctor and thus have a fairly small long-term-care population. Still, during those six weeks, I had over seventy people sent to the hospital. Most were sent for falls, confusion, high blood pressure, abnormal labs, or breathing problems. More than half were admitted to the hospital, but in my estimation only a handful of those really needed in-hospital treatment. Many returned with infections, were functionally and mentally more impaired, and were no better off than they had been before in regard to the problem for which they were sent. Virtually all of them, even those only spending time in the emergency room, had thousands of dollars of testing and treatment that resolved nothing. Even with the most conservative estimates of fees, the overall cost to Medicare for hospital visits for this six-week slice of my small practice was several hundreds of thousands of dollars. And the cost to the patients, to their quality of life and their functional capacity, was immeasurable.

In our county, certain "hot spots" have been identified in which the hospitalization rate is high. These are small geographical areas where substantially more people find themselves in the hospital regularly than anywhere else in the county. What unites the hot spots of Howard County is that each of them has a long-term-care facility within its boundaries, which is where the bulk of hospital admissions originate. Ironically, since I am affiliated with many long-term-care institutions in the county, I am likely targeted as a doctor who overutilizes the hospital simply by the hot-spot equation. Thus, despite the fact that I aggressively keep people out of the hospital with as much power as I possess, that power pales in comparison with the forces in long-term care pushing patients in the other direction. Some reformers believe that I can alter that reality, that if facilities are better educated, that if they call us every time something goes wrong, that if we have a nurse practitioner or doctor available to drive over there at a moment's notice, then hospitalizations can be averted. But that myth flies in the face of the reality of regulations, finances, and attitude. Doctors and nurses do not want to hospitalize the frail elderly, and many families deep in their hearts do not want to either, but the system pushes the aggressive option on us anyway.

Given the reality of patient and family wishes that favor palliation, one wonders why the current trends cannot be reversed. Ninety-six percent of family members report that comfort is their primary goal. But as one researcher states: "The pattern of transition among nursing home residents with advanced cognitive impairment is often inconsistent with that goal." A fifth of nursing-home residents with dementia are sent to the hospital, and in some states that number is closer to 40 percent. There is no correlation between patient/family wishes and the number of hospital trips.[13] In another study, 25 percent of long-term-care residents were hospitalized at least once during a six-month interval, without correlation to patient/family wishes to avoid hospitalization. "Physically frail patients, who may be the least likely to benefit from hospitalizations, are the most likely to be hospitalized," the study concluded.[14] In another study, 40 percent of hospitalizations occurred within three months of nursing-home admission, and the rate of hospitalization was 566 per 1,000 residents a year.[15]

An aggressive mentality sprouts early in a resident's nursing-home stay and can grow as time moves forward and signs of illness manifest. When staff and physicians/NPs have time to discuss the futility of thorough care and the natural decline inherent to aging with patients and families, a small dent can be made in the trend. Facilities with more doctors and nurse practitioners available to see residents and families have fewer hospitalizations, although even those numbers are high.[16] But many patients and families have not pondered these issues before marching into long-term care, and then are stuck by an atmosphere that pushes them in a direction that may not reflect their wishes. Only 75 percent of adults even have advanced directives,[17] and many of those who have completed living wills have done so in a vacuum where they could not envision many of the decisions they now face. In my state, every resident admitted to a long-term-care facility must complete a MOLST (medical orders for life-sustaining treatment) form, which is essentially a living will, and for many this is the first time they have pondered such weighty questions. Financial realities and state surveys are two other prime reasons that hospitalization occurs with such high frequency.[18] Families are often blindsided by the long-term-care onslaught, although many, too, have some degree of faith in thorough medical care, which allows them to acquiesce to what is transpiring.

Hospice

Among the elderly, palliative approaches can decrease pain, shortness of breath, and general discomfort while increasing quality of life as well as patient and family satisfaction. There is no proven increased mortality in the elderly population who chose to be palliative. But the idea of hospice and palliative care is frightening to many patients and families. They believe that by accepting comfort care they have to abandon hope and accept that death is inevitable. Such a misconception of palliative care is embedded in Medicare's regulations, since Medicare rules stipulate that people have to be end of life and relinquish disease treatment in order to obtain palliative benefits by enrolling in hospice.[19] In other words, Medicare will pay for palliative care only if a patient is on the verge of death.

Thus to most players in long-term care—from providers to administrators to families and patients—the only responsible and financially feasible alternative to excessive care that leads so frequently to hospitalization is that of giving up and preparing for death. Recently I was confronted by a facility nurse forcing me to make a bitter decision that has become quite familiar to me. One of my patients, who has severe dementia and is unstable, fell and hit his head. The facility wanted to send him to the hospital, but his daughter did not want that done. She had come to the conclusion that she wanted her dad to be comfortable. So the nurses told me that the daughter had a choice: either send her dad to the hospital or enroll him in hospice. This black-and-white option is something that is thrust at doctors and families almost every day. And at its core is an assumption that if families reject the ethos of aggressive care and hospitalization, then their only other choice is to let their loved one die.

Hospice is a Medicare benefit designed to help people at the end of life, typically for those who have cancer and who are actively dying. Hospice patients can obtain more nursing, extra support, pain medicines, medical equipment, and even a brief stay in a hospice inpatient unit when death is imminent and needs are extensive. Typically patients can receive care in the comfort of their homes or long-term-care facilities, fully paid for by Medicare. Hospice provides emotional and physical support. Anyone who has been part of hospice, either as a family member or health-care provider, agrees that it is the most wonderful experience they could have had during the most difficult time of their lives. In my experience, hospice has been one of the most forward-thinking and compassionate programs that Medicare ever devised, allowing people to die with dignity and without stress, paying for home care and for appropriate treatments without delay or administrative hurdles, and keeping people out of harm's way when they are most vulnerable. I am lucky to work with several excellent hospice agencies that provide superb care.

While hospice, when appropriately used, helps residents in long-term care die in comfort, hospice can also be something employed by facilities and families as the only crutch they have to keep residents away from aggressive care and to have Medicare foot some of the bill. Once families agree to hospice they essentially declare that they want only comfort and are prepared for death. The hospice agency gets paid quite well by Medicare to provide such a benefit, about $4,700 per month per enrollee.[20] One *New York Times* report examined the enrollment of patients in hospice and found that many remained in hospice care for prolonged periods of time, sometimes requiring no or minimal services. During those stints hospice was paid $147–$856/day ($4,410/month–$25,680/month) depending on the level of care and "regardless of whether a hospice actually provides service."[21] A more recent *Washington Post* exposé made a similar claim, reporting that the number of patients discharged alive from hospice increased by 50 percent between 2002–2012, with an increased average length of stay during that period. The article's authors state that a large number of these patients were not hospice appropriate, and were enrolled only because of the financial remuneration.[22] Perhaps many of these patients were not on the verge of death, but they did not want excessive care. With hospice, they could achieve their goals and get some financial help. Without hospice, hospitalization often becomes the only recourse, since home care and appropriate long-term care are not financially feasible otherwise under Medicare. And perhaps, too, some of these patients actually clinically improved after being enrolled in hospice, living longer because they were removed from the claws of aggressive care, such as Mrs. S who I discussed earlier.

In many long-term-care facilities, then, hospice is a way for the facility to get an albatross off its neck. If a family does not buy into the mentality of aggressive care that is expected and assumed, then the family is advised to enroll their loved one in hospice. Once a patient is in hospice, then the facility no longer bears the responsibility to prevent and account for their decline.

Certainly, that is not the intent of hospice, but for many families and facilities it is the only palliative option Medicare provides. I always say that the landscape between hospice and aggression is called good geriatric care. This is ground rarely trod because it is something Medicare does not support financially, even though hospice agencies would be ideal vehicles to oversee the delivery of such care. Palliative care, as we have discussed, does not assume that patients are on the verge of death. Rather, it correctly reasons that with medical care focused on comfort and dignity that relies less on number chasing and testing, quality improves for patient and family alike. It is the basic soul of good geriatric health care, especially for the old and frail residents of long-term-care facilities. It is the type of care that many hospice agencies would like to deliver if only they could be authorized to do so, and it comes likely at a much lower cost.

Hospice is certainly problematic in several ways, most of which stem from Medicare's suffocating rules. Patients can turn hospice on and off at will. They can discharge themselves from hospice and rush to the hospital to get aggressive treatment, followed by a "skilled" rehabilitation stay, and then return to hospice subsequently. They can also continue to see specialists and maintain full code status. Therefore, there is no need for hospice patients to truly adhere to a palliative mind-set since Medicare will pay either way. Also, because of its function as an instrument in end-of-life care, hospice relies heavily on pain management, something not necessarily relevant to the needs of many elderly with dementia. But most problematic about hospice is its narrow focus. Because admission to hospice is becoming more restrictive, many patients who would benefit from a palliative approach do not qualify. By stipulating that hospice can serve only end-of-life patients, Medicare is denying palliative treatment to a large number of elders who would benefit from such an approach, and as such is inflicting financial harm on itself by opening the door to expensive and ineffective aggressive care.

Looking Ahead

The future of long-term care is not necessarily any rosier than what we are seeing now, although Medicare is trying to make some changes, as we will explore in the next chapter. At a recent conference of medical directors (AMDA) held in Maryland, I caught a glimpse of what may lie ahead. Talks by academic leaders, CMS officials, and influential medical directors spelled out a frightening scenario. Long-term-care regulations not only are here to stay, but they may become more intense, especially in assisted-living facilities. Penalties for doctors and facilities are escalating, and surveys will likely occur with increasing frequency. Privacy laws (HIPAA) are becoming more tightly regulated in long-term care, leading to more possible fines for facilities and doctors alike. And the very ethos of aggressive treatment seemed to have gained a foothold in this group of wise geriatric doctors, many of whom spoke about the need to tightly control disease among the frail elderly.

At one of the talks, a group of geriatric leaders from major academic institutions outlined a possible nursing home of the future. One of them talked about how nursing homes may soon be able to offer blood transfusions, aggressive treatments, minor surgeries, and even a hospital level of treatment. In other words, they would keep nursing-home residents out of the hospital by essentially transforming nursing homes into hospitals.[23] Somehow reformers have convinced themselves that providing aggressive and intensive care to the frail elderly within the nursing-home walls is good medicine. In the end, long-term care seems to mimic a hospital more every day. Unfortunately, its population is the one most hurt by a hospital level of care.

Current reforms by CMS hope to curb hospitalization, seemingly the most obvious and costly ramification of aggressive care. Medicare programs give some indications that alternatives to the three-night rule are being considered, although nothing concrete has been proposed to replace it. One informed speaker at the AMDA conference told us that the three-night rule was here to stay, so I am not convinced that its end is near. More saliently, Medicare is looking closely at skilled nursing-home residents, devising plans that financially reward and punish hospitals and nursing homes that readmit skilled residents to the hospital within thirty days of their hospital discharge. CMS reasons that substantial cost is incurred by such readmissions. But the program is not without its flaws. Because CMS has handed hospitals the power to administer the global funds to cover the first thirty days of a skilled stay, nursing homes are left in the cold. Very likely hospitals will start building their own subacute units so they can better control the post-hospital window, and this will take from nursing homes their most profitable residents. Also, while Medicare's thirty-day readmission moratorium dissuades facilities from hospitalizing a select group of residents for a brief stretch of time, its payment structure continues to encourage admission outside that window. In fact, for hospitals and nursing homes to reap any financial incentives that Medicare will provide them to avert readmissions, there must first be an initial hospital admission to initiate the process, an irony that obfuscates the program's purpose.

Can nursing homes really prevent hospital readmissions in the current environment? How can one group of residents (skilled patients in the thirty-day window) be treated one way, and all other residents (where hospitalization may be beneficial to the nursing home and hospital alike) be treated differently? Can the modus operandi be turned on and off for different groups of patients that quickly? Also, during that thirty-day window, nursing homes will still be subjected to the same regulations and threats of lawsuits that make aggressive care and hospitalization seem necessary, and thus they can be hurt just as much from not hospitalizing a resident as from hospitalizing her.

As long as the current long-term-care culture remains intact, reform will be nothing but window dressing on one of the most counterproductive drains of Medicare funds. Without malpractice reform, regulatory reform, and profound alterations of Medicare's payment structure, including the elimination of the three-day rule, long-term-care facilities have no realistic capacity to move toward a medically sensible and economically sound mode of care. Facilities do want to make that leap, but their hands are tied. As we conclude the book, we will discuss current reform efforts and explore other ideas that may help save Medicare from its current quagmire.

6

QUALITY AND VALUE

Moving toward a Cure

We now have a vast and costly health-care industry devoted to finding and responding to turtles [conditions that if left alone would cause no harm]. Our ever more sensitive technologies turn up more and more abnormalities—cancers, clogged arteries, damaged-looking knees and backs—that aren't actually causing problems and never will. And then we doctors try to fix them, even though the result is often more harm than good. . . . An entire health-care system has been devoted to this game. Yet we're finally seeing evidence that the system can change—even in the most expensive places for health care in the country.

ATUL GAWANDE, "Overkill," May 2015

In January 2015 Health and Human Services Secretary Sylvia Burwell announced that Medicare would be shifting its paradigm. Rather than paying physicians and hospitals for episodic visits, it would be reimbursing them based on the quality and value of their work. According to Burwell: "Today's announcement is about improving the quality of care we receive when we are sick, while at the same time spending our health care dollars more wisely. We believe these goals can drive transformative change, help us manage and track progress, and create accountability for measurable improvement. . . . New targets have been set for value-based payment: 85% of Medicare fee-for-service payments should be tied to quality or value by 2016, and 30% of Medicare payments should be tied to quality or value through alternative payment models by 2016 (50% by 2018)."[1] In April Congress passed a final "doc fix" law that prevented further cuts in physician payment, reiterating that its long-term goal is to tie reimbursement to quality and value.

But how do we define quality and value? In this book we have discussed Medicare's definition of what constitutes quality, something that has been inscribed in their quality indicators to which physicians have been compelled to adhere. To Medicare, quality can be generically defined, quantified, and easily measured. As we have shown, Medicare's quality indicators often fail to measure true geriatric quality, while leading to overtesting and overtreatment and preventing doctors and patients from having meaningful conversations that lead to shared decision making. Is this the quality to which Secretary Burwell and Congress are referring? "Value," too, has a nebulous meaning. Does it imply that doctors will be rewarded by saving the system money, or by cutting services, or by having patients who are less risky? Will doctors who care for the frailest elderly, or for "noncompliant" patients who gravitate to the hospital, be punished if their patients exhaust more resources than the patients of a doctor who looks after a younger and healthier population?

In April 2015 President Obama signed a bipartisan Medicare reform bill that linked pay to performance. Doctors will soon be rated on a scale of 0–100 based on their "quality" and "value" scorecards, with a large portion of physician pay being based on that scale. But even though the program is slated to start in 2019, no one has yet definitively stated how such terms will be defined. According to David Blumenthal of the Commonwealth Fund, which sponsors health-policy research, attempts to rate medical interventions have "unleashed a multitude of uncoordinated, inconsistent, and often duplicative measurement and reporting initiatives." Some initiatives that use metrics to improve care have done just the opposite, and most measures that are being utilized to rate doctors have no proof of efficacy to back them up. Says Ann Greiner from the National Quality Forum, which sets standards for health-care metrics: "If you're going to link payment to a measure, you want to make sure that that measure is reliable and valid and can improve care."[2] Currently, the guidelines are not only inaccurate but are also geared toward population health, and thus may well have no relevance to the individual patient who is sitting in front of me at any moment. In fact, many measures, if instituted, would be either detrimental to many of my patients, or may be something that my patient chooses not to accept after we discuss it. Thus, by following good geriatric care, and listening to my patients after conversing about the pros and cons of medical interventions, my pay may be cut by our new performance-focused model of health care.

Ultimately, until society, and Medicare, can adequately define quality and value and individualize them, then no reform effort will be successful. Society has already reached a verdict regarding what constitutes thorough medical care, and it is unlikely that most Americans are simply going to abandon their notion that quality often equals aggressive care. In theory, Americans criticize the huge expenditures being injected into the Medicare system, and resent paying more taxes to cover those costs. Both political parties agree that we must curtail wasteful spending. But, because of what I call the Katrina effect, most people are opposed in theory to government waste, but demand that government spending be provided to them when they think they need it ASAP! Much as many Louisiana political leaders opposed wasteful spending by the federal government before and after Katrina (including voting against funds for Hurricane Sandy) while demanding instant and extensive federal funds when a hurricane struck their shores, Americans expect and demand unrestricted medical care when they have a medical problem, even if they are opposed to Medicare's wasteful expenditures. Part of that expectation derives from the false notion of what constitutes thorough care, something that is incessantly being pumped into the public psyche by the press.

Consider, for example, press coverage of the placement of a stent in one of President George W. Bush's heart's blood vessels. Apparently, during his annual physical, his very thorough primary-care doctor ordered an exercise stress test, which demonstrated an abnormality. President Bush then had a CT angiogram, followed by a cardiac catheterization and stent of the blocked vessel. The news media trumpeted the medical "save" orchestrated by President Bush's outstanding doctor. One NPR program marveled at our former president's care, stating that other patients should demand similar thorough treatment.

But, as a well-reasoned opinion piece in the *Washington Post* argued, President Bush's stress test was likely unnecessary and was potentially harmful. The physician authors stated: "If Mr. Bush had visited a general internist practicing sound, evidence-based care, he would not have had cardiac testing." At age sixty-seven, our former president jogged regularly and bicycled long distances all without symptoms or limitations. No study has demonstrated the efficacy of screening stress tests in such a patient, nor has any study shown that stenting the type of occluded artery found during the testing improves either lifespan or life quality. In fact, now President Bush will be at higher risk for having to take two blood thinners to prevent the stent from collapsing and blocking the vessel entirely.[3] Most significantly, President Bush now carries a diagnosis of coronary artery disease (CAD), a label that will define him for the rest of his life; lead to more tests, procedures, medicines, and specialist visits down the road; and may even impact him psychologically. Worse still, while it is unclear whether Medicare would pay for the initial stress test given to President Bush and patients like him, it certainly would pay for all subsequent testing and the placement of the stent, and it would continue to pay for all cardiac testing, specialist visits, and further stenting for as long as our president, or any other Medicare recipient, lives. One test ordered in the name of "thorough" set off a cascade of further testing and treatments, all without proven benefit, all with potential harm, and yet Medicare paid without blinking an eye, and most of the news media praised the wonderful medical care.

President Bush is only sixty-seven. Many of my patients who are much older certainly have blocked arteries. If we look hard enough we will find them, and we can send them, too, on a similar expensive and precarious course financed by Medicare and cheered by society and the lay press. But we also have evidence that such aggressive treatment often is not medically beneficial to our oldest patients, and may actually be deleterious. Even as our society scoffs at the high cost of Medicare, it ignores the simple fact that Medicare is enabling and even encouraging our costly trek through a wilderness of inappropriate medical care for the frail elderly.

The Katrina effect has a profound impact on Medicare reform efforts and is the primary reason that rationing is such a bedeviled word. We know that stenting may be excessively performed and is enriching certain doctors, but we demand the stent for ourselves when the doctor says we need one, and we truly believe that the stent has saved our lives. Also, many Americans believe that since they have put money into Medicare during their working lives, they deserve all the medical care they desire; after all, they paid for that care. Unfortunately, since the average American spends $387,000 of Medicare money during his/her lifetime, and has only contributed $88,000 to Medicare,[4] society is paying for the vast majority of the excessive and wasteful care that Medicare is both allowing and encouraging.

Perhaps we can redefine the thorough care that older people truly seek. Perhaps, if given reasonable options, many patients would follow a different path, one that leads to better medical outcomes at lower cost and with improved satisfaction. Part of what hampers a sensible health-care delivery system is the perception—often trumpeted by the press and by many members of the medical establishment—that more tests and treatments and drugs will lead to optimal outcomes. Patients and doctors lack access to actual risk-benefit analysis of medical interventions and are fed a copious platter of contrived (relative risk-benefit) data that prevents them from making rational and shared medical decisions. But even more significantly, Medicare—through its clinical practice guidelines and payment structures—pushes patients and doctors down a precarious road that ultimately derives mediocre results at substantially high cost and with poor patient/doctor satisfaction with the process and outcome. If we want to make the system work, we must profoundly alter the soul and mechanics of Medicare.

What Does Work

To determine what will work, we need to look at systems that have a proven success record, both home and abroad. Many medical economists and thinkers look to Europe for solutions, since their care is objectively superior to ours at a much lower cost. In our own country, we do have a government-financed health-care system that provides nontraditional models of care and yet produces excellent health outcomes and high patient satisfaction for some of the sickest patients in the system. This is our Department of Veterans Affairs (VA), where patients have limited specialty access, ample primary care, a strict drug formulary, and services geared to help the specific patient population being served.[5] The VA is certainly not free of its own difficulties, not the least of which are a growing reliance on clinical performance measures and a shortage of primary-care doctors at times (leading to longer wait times, something endemic to the primary-care shortage that grips our entire nation), but it achieves quality care for patients at a low cost. Also, the VA is always innovating. With expansive home-care services, specialty consultations that do not require a visit, and the ability of doctors to "visit" patients at their homes through telephone and computer technology, the VA is able to achieve its goals without having to resort to as much specialization and hospitalization. Medicare, with its strict rules about paying doctors primarily for face-to-face visits and procedures, will not permit this efficient and effective model of care.

Another innovative strategy that has been enacted in this country for several decades relies on capitated health-care plans called health maintenance organizations (HMOs). Medicare HMOs are insurance companies of varying sizes that are paid a specified global fee by Medicare per patient (capitation) and are expected to take full care of that patient—including all hospitalizations, doctor visits, and procedures—for that amount of money. If the companies can treat their cohort of patients for less money than Medicare pays them, they win financially. If not, they lose. Therefore, HMOs work hard to provide sensible, efficient care.

Unfortunately, HMOs have not made a significant dent in our Medicare crisis. During their history HMOs have proven to be unpopular among many patients because they are perceived as restricting patient choice,[6] thus implying that they ration care. Therefore, they have tended to attract the healthiest patients who spend the least amount of health-care dollars. Also, studies have demonstrated that HMOs do not curtail doctor visits, or even reduce the cost of end-of-life care.[7] Probably the most significant limitation of managed care is that it has never had enough traction to really make an impact. Now more Medicare HMOs are emerging, but under the ACA the current 14 percent subsidy that Medicare pays to HMO vendors will be eliminated, leaving Medicare HMOs with an uncertain future.

While working at a retirement community I had the opportunity to be part of an HMO that was constructed and piloted by the primary-care physicians of the community. It was never a large endeavor, and I was not privy to whether it achieved real financial success even with Medicare's 14 percent subsidy, but from my perspective it did work. We eliminated the three-day rule, allowing us to treat patients in our nursing home and in their homes without resorting to hospitalization. Nurses followed patients at home, and primary-care doctors made most crucial decisions. Patients still had unfettered access to specialists, tests were not restricted, and clinical practice guidelines retained too much importance, but compared to standard Medicare, the HMO did allow us to take care of our patients in a more humane, sensible fashion. Hospitalization rates dropped dramatically, and both patient and physician satisfaction were higher. Any model for health-care reform should reflect what we have learned from HMOs, whether done through Medicare Advantage Plans (that allow local control of funds) or in Medicare itself.

Atul Gawande, in his article "Overkill," highlights a successful primary-care group called WellMed, operating mostly in Texas and Florida, that allows its doctors more time and resources to take care of patients, leading to dramatic reductions in hospitalization and testing, and better outcomes and satisfaction. Like with the VA system and the HMO in which I worked, this primary-care-based method has achieved better health care at lower cost for the sickest and most vulnerable patients.[8] It is difficult to determine if groups such as WellMed will be as successful once they are more generalized, and it is troubling that they, like the VA and many HMOs, are relying on far too many clinical guidelines to measure success, thus homogenizing care in a way that can be deleterious to the elderly and frustrating for doctor and patient alike, as we have discussed. But the crux of all of these successful strategies is to focus on primary care and enable the primary-care doctor to have ample time to actually engage with his/her patient in a meaningful way. Steven Schimpff, in his excellent book on primary care, *Fixing the Primary Care Crisis,* shows definitively that when primary-care doctors have more time to care for their patients and can focus on each one individually, every measure of success is enhanced: quality care, cost of care, and satisfaction. He cites many examples of systems that have implemented that strategy with positive results.[9]

Reformers are also employing a strategy, used by some local hospitals and insurance systems today, that focuses on education to reduce hospitalization. For those patients hospitalized frequently or who spend large amounts of money for their care, care coordinators will help them navigate the medical landscape. Social workers and nurses will guide such patients through the health-care-delivery system, assisting them with doctor appointments, self-care, and education. Some small studies have shown a cost savings from such a model, as well as a reduction in hospital readmission in the first thirty days after discharge.[10] A more recent and extensive $300 million program, funded by CMS and the ACA, awarding community groups funds to cut down on hospital readmissions has largely failed. Only four out of forty-eight groups dropped readmissions, and the majority of groups dropped out of the program entirely.[11] Because such programs are in their infancy, their true utility is yet to be seen.

Currently many reformers absorb the lesson of HMOs and other successful programs and reach what I believe to be an erroneous conclusion. They assume that if physicians are paid for their performance rather than for each visit and procedure, then physicians will be incented to provide more efficient, low-cost care and keep elderly patients out of the hospital. This approach is rife with problems. It assumes that physicians can influence the specific care that their patients pursue, even if patients are intent on leaping onto the "thorough" train and are often pushed in that direction. Specialization, the threat of lawsuits, long-term-care regulations, and a belief among Americans that more care is better care all will not simply disappear under a pay-for-performance approach. Thus, unless primary-care doctors can impact the aggressive medical environment in which we all live, we cannot alter the course our patients pursue. Currently, pay-for-performance models try to nudge doctors to do the "right" thing without giving them the tools to carry out that objective. What enabled our small HMO to succeed is that we wrote our own rules, we could treat people at home, and we were able to spend Medicare's money in ways that make sense for our patients.

In addition, it is very unclear how performance will be defined under a pay-for-performance model. Under proposed systems, physician performance is typically defined by clinical performance measures, which, as we have discussed, do not reflect true quality geriatric care. If we aggressively treat diabetes, control blood pressure, treat heart-disease patients with statins, order bone-density tests, and allow open access to specialty care, then our performance is deemed to be of high quality. Thus, those of us who practice good geriatric care, and who talk to our patients about the actual risks and benefits of certain medical interventions, are going to be labeled poor performers under any system using clinical guidelines. Also, performance is defined by how much money our patients cost the system, something completely out of our control.

Another idea being tossed around is to push the Medicare eligibility age up to sixty-seven. The thought is that by eliminating a few years of Medicare enrollees from the insurance market, Medicare can instantly save money. But such a concept ignores what we know about both the demographics of aging and the projected spending pattern of Medicare recipients. Most of Medicare's money is spent on our oldest citizens, a group of people whose numbers are expanding rapidly. In fact, the cost savings by denying younger Medicare patients access to insurance would barely put a dent in our pending Medicare crisis given that most of Medicare's funds are spent on the frailest elderly who are the least likely to benefit from aggressive care. In addition, pulling health insurance away from a vulnerable population is certainly not an effective means of assuring optimal outcomes. Thus, rather than alter the age of eligibility, the goal of reform should be to improve care for all Medicare recipients, perhaps relying on programs that have already demonstrated at least some degree of success.

Medicare Reform and the ACA

Currently multiple reform efforts are being proposed and instituted to help save Medicare from its accelerating spiral of financial peril. Many are emanating from the government through Medicare's "innovation center"[12] and the Affordable Care Act (ACA).[13] As a practicing physician I have been bombarded by a host of new rules and regulations. Some are so poorly explained to me that I am forced to pay consultants to walk me through the process. Some are so poorly executed that they simply are not possible to carry out. I have been to conferences, read articles, and have talked to CMS experts in an effort to stay one step ahead, often to no avail. This year we hired a full-time employee whose only job is to implement and assure compliance with Medicare's novel programs, requirements, and rules.

One example of a new cost-saving measure is Medicare's assault on home health and home medical equipment, both of which help keep my patients out of the hospital and away from aggressive care, but both of which have been overutilized and have led to well-documented unnecessary spending. Unfortunately, while the intention of reformers in this regard is sensible given the history of fraud and abuse in home health, the strategy of curtailing home care actually may lead to more cost and a higher hospitalization rate. For me, it has thwarted my ability to deliver appropriate low-cost care that many of my patients seek. Medicare currently pays only for very limited services at home for brief durations, and the home-health nurses with whom I work talk about copious new restrictions that limit the scope of what they can do for my older patients. For me, I now have tremendous paperwork requirements to initiate and retain home-health services and to order home medical equipment, especially more expensive items such as electric wheelchairs (which still cost Medicare less than a day in the hospital) and even manual wheelchairs and hospital beds. I now spend over an hour a day filling out the pile of forms that are tossed on my desk primarily related to home health and medical equipment. While the burdens of paperwork have accentuated for home care, I have encountered no such barriers to sending patients to hospitals or specialists and ordering expensive tests. Those remain easy to execute under the ACA and Medicare!

The financial burden to our practice from government-initiated regulations and reforms like the new home-health rules has been substantial. But other measures are even more costly. For instance, to comply with the electronic-medical-record requirement we have had to pay for increasingly costly software, pay an IT expert to provide ongoing services, and set up expensive security measures, as well as buy computers and hardware with regularity. (Ironically, too, our paper costs have also escalated in our paperless EMR system!) Also, given that there is understandable speculation in the medical community that some of the ACA will be financed by auditing doctor offices and fining those whose billing and charting practices do not comply with Medicare standards,[14] I have taken out both coding and HIPAA insurance plans, both of which are costly. Although I believe I am coding correctly and do not commit HIPAA violations, I can easily envision an auditor finding a few subjective problems that could cost our practice tens of thousands of dollars in fines, if not more.

Recently my HIPAA and coding insurer dropped me, citing the fact that auditors (who are paid a certain percentage of the fines they levy on doctors, giving them great incentive to escalate the fines) are now targeting geriatric doctors who care for patients in long-term-care facilities or who make home visits. I immediately wrote to my congressman and senators.

I expressed my outrage at the ACA, a bill I supported, but which now seemed to be strangling geriatric care. I cited the cost and fear of audits, the cost of electronic records, the increasing regulatory burdens of HIPAA and of required adherence to copious clinical guidelines that are often irrelevant to our patients, the increasing paperwork and the inability to provide patients with home health care and with simple medical equipment, the introduction of new billing codes (ICD-10) that are burdensome and time-consuming, and the incessant threat of arbitrary reimbursement cuts coupled with a demand for more accountability. My congressman's staffer did call me back, and we spoke a few times; she seemed sympathetic but was not optimistic that there would be change.

Several weeks later our practice was audited. We were asked to provide forty charts to a CMS contractor. Our sin: that we billed too many codes for seeing people in assisted-living facilities, where many of our patients reside. I spoke to people in CMS, to consultants, to insurance brokers. We read through the forty charts to assess whether we had documented everything correctly. We knew that even one missing line from the CMS template would be considered fraud. Although most of the notes seemed extensively documented, none were perfect, and anything less than perfect is potentially considered overpayment. The process was frightening and time-consuming. In the end we came through with flying colors, but we also know that more audits lie ahead. In fact, only six months later, I was again audited, this time targeting my use of electronic medical records. With all the extraneous work and cost Medicare's reforms have created for us, it seems that Medicare has decided that it is easier to assault small geriatric primary-care practices than to have the resolve to fix a broken system.

We in primary care no longer receive the 10 percent bonus to our Medicare revenue that was designed to boost our income and pay for the cost of many reforms that have raised our overhead, although we can receive additional bonuses if we comply with electronic-medical-record standards and participate in our ACO (which we will discuss). But what we have had to pay to adhere to the increasing regulations and punitive audits being carried out in the name of innovative reform wipes out any possible fiscal help being given to us. None of this is helping to make primary care a more attractive field, and from what I can see none of it will make any dent in Medicare's pending financial collapse or in our ability to care for elderly patients.

The dearth of primary care, and the explosion of specialization in our medical society, have led to a procedure-oriented culture that is sucking Medicare's funds away without providing any proven medical benefits, something even more apparent for the oldest of our patients. Nothing in Medicare's reforms is changing that reality. The income of procedure-oriented specialists has increased dramatically over the past decade, while primary-care income has inched up modestly, something typically erased by the increased regulatory burdens to which we are forced to adhere. Dermatologists, who perform the biopsies we discussed in a past chapter, previously earned an income similar to primary-care doctors, but now are the fourth-highest paid specialty and have one of the lightest workloads according to the *Times* article I cited. In my opinion, primary care has the opposite profile: the lowest paid, and one of the highest workloads. Despite the talk of government reform and the promises of the ACA, aggressive, specialized medicine will continue to dominate the medical landscape as long as it is well compensated and is not discouraged. Reform cannot work as long as we live in a society that thrives on excess. The fact that Congress has cut primary-care salaries at the very time that the government is dropping a tremendous load of regulations, time-consuming requirements that squander time for doctor-patient discourse during visits, audits, technological cost, and a confusing array of rules on the laps of primary-care doctors suggests that, despite lipservice to the contrary, Medicare's masters have no intention of helping improve primary care in this country or changing our specialty-oriented health care delivery system in any profound way.

I will discuss a few of the government-sponsored reforms that have arrived or are on the way. For those readers less interested in the minutia of current reform efforts, you can skip to the next section, "Trying a Different Approach." I will say that I know many people, doctors and others, who work in CMS trying to make Medicare sensible and financially solvent. Their ideas are often quite bold, and they do comprehend many of the issues that thwart Medicare's ability to carry out its primary mission in helping the elderly. But politics, bureaucracy, and vested interests hamper even the most idealistic reformer's efforts to apply pragmatic repairs to what we all know is a broken system. Within the tight boundaries of their roles in CMS, many reformers have started to script some fixes, some of which have not been successful in the eyes of a primary-care doctor like me, and others that perhaps do have some potential.

Electronic Medical Records

I have worked with Electronic Medical Records (EMRs) for well over a decade, and began my new practice with computers, laptops, and medical software. Without a doubt, the EMR caused me more stress and consternation during my first year in solo practice than anything else. After spending weeks setting up the system, it continuously crashed, always at the least opportune times. I used to stay up past midnight completing my notes and fighting a system that refused to cooperate. After a great waste of dollars and time, and after consulting various experts who often only made matters worse, we stabilized our medical record system, although we still have serious problems on a regular basis. So much can go wrong that likely it will; but after so many years of regular crashes and Internet failures we have finally accommodated to it. It is still where most of us squander the bulk of our time and overhead. We are typically in front of the computer more than we are in front of our patients, and even when we are with patients we are focused on typing our scripted notes in exactly the format Medicare demands of us, something that clearly distracts from the doctor-patient encounter.

Medicare does pay for us to certify our medical records, but the stipend, while substantial (approximately $20,000 for initial certification, less incrementally later), costs us a great deal of time, money, and frustration. I spent approximately forty hours completing the many checklists that CMS mandates to prove my compliance with its EMR requirement, and that is for only part 1 of the process. The Medicare stipend does not come close to paying all the expenses that go into initiating and maintaining an EMR. Technology is our biggest overhead cost, other than salaries. From a patient standpoint, EMRs are not well accepted; they cause doctors to stare at a screen and madly type on a keyboard rather than looking into a patient's eyes and listen to what they are saying. In fact, we doctors have no choice; unless we type our notes as Medicare dictates, and unless we enter into the computer all of the many necessary ingredients that the purveyors of quality have demanded of us, then we are vulnerable to salary reduction and reprimand. A typical note takes me fifteen minutes to complete outside of my time with the patient. And I am a good typist! Clearly, my ability to converse with the patient is impaired by the EMR, something not lost on my patients and their families. One of my patients thought I had a nervous tick in my hand because it was constantly banging on the keyboard. Many of my patients have asked me to stop typing and to look at them, something I simply cannot do.

Medicare and the ACA both tout EMRs as crucial to health-care reform. Perhaps in the future EMRs will help us all be connected: doctor to doctor, doctor to hospital, patient to doctor, lab to doctor and patient. Little of that is occurring now, and with HIPAA hovering over all of us like a voracious vulture, I cannot imagine connectivity being a very substantial force in the near future. So at this point, EMRs allow us to write notes, send prescriptions, and print/fax orders, that is all. In 2015 all participating Medicare physicians were required to have an EMR, and unless we "prove" we are using EMRs "meaningfully" we will be subjected to reimbursement cuts and likely audits, as happened already to me. Proving meaningful use tacks on about an hour of frivolous work to my typical day, as I type information into the computer that Medicare demands of me but which is not clinically relevant.

How successful are EMRs? They have saved the VA system money. But in the world of private practice, no such financial benefit has been seen. A 2005 RAND study predicted that EMRs may save the system $81 billion annually. By 2013, however, no health-care savings have yet occurred. In fact, some suggest that EMRs actually increase test ordering and thus cost.[15] They also allow doctors to increase the billing for their services and possibly charge more for visits. And of course, they divert physician time and resources away from patient care and toward note-taking and data entry. Likely the EMRs will be an important component of modern medicine, but at this juncture they are neither helping the quality of geriatric care nor saving the system money. In fact, they are really just very sophisticated headaches!

Physician Quality Reporting System (PQRS)

An important mission of CMS is to ensure that Medicare doctors practice "quality" geriatric care, as we have discussed. PQRS is simply a means of persuading Medicare physicians to adhere to a specified set of clinical guidelines. When CMS built its PQRS system, it offered a small incentive to those who complied. Now physicians suffer reimbursement cuts if they do not comply. Quality is measured by many parameters, and physicians can dig deep into websites and thick books to find specific clinical-practice guidelines that can be followed and documented electronically to satisfy Medicare's PQRS requirement. Each year the number of measures with which we have to comply grows, and we have to generate new notes in our computer to prove our compliance to auditors, as well as spending more of our office-visit time inquiring about and documenting these measures.

Under the current quality parameters laid out by Medicare and the ACA, certain doctors will be rewarded: a doctor who puts her elderly patients on multiple blood-pressure medicines that drive their pressures down to "normal" levels, causing them more confusion and fatigue, and leading one of them to fall and break a hip; a doctor who insists his patients get bone-density tests, mammograms, and colonoscopies without discussing them with their patients; a doctor who tells patients with afib that they have no choice but to be on Coumadin; a doctor who stares at the computer and types endlessly without listening to his patients. Other doctors will be punished: those who spend too much time talking with their patients, who offer patients options and ultimately listen to their patients' wishes, who back off on tests and medicines when they have adverse clinical impact on their patients or when their patients choose other options, who spend visits discussing issues that are important to their patients rather than checking off clinical guidelines.

While I laud CMS for trying to enhance quality, I am not quite sure how this particular reform measure will help improve real geriatric quality, especially given the parameters by which we are being judged. In fact, many of us in primary care cite Medicare's quality indicator requirements as one of the most wasteful and time-consuming endeavors in which we are being forced to participate. Also, early data would suggest that performance payment will not be as substantial as originally stated. In a large demonstration project where one thousand physician groups were offered enhanced payments for following clinical guidelines, only fourteen groups (1.4%) were deemed to have achieved sufficient quality to be awarded a bonus.[16] Thus the reality of using quality indicators to gauge physician performance and rewarding doctors in a meaningful way seems fleeting at best.

Accountable Care Organizations (ACOs)

Perhaps the most promising, if perplexing, concept created by the ACA are ACOs, voluntary HMO-like entities that doctors and/or institutions join in an effort to cut cost and improve quality. The basic premise of ACOs is to encourage doctors and hospitals to combine forces and utilize care coordination, clinical practice guidelines, and enhanced communication to decrease the wasteful consumption of care. The ACO will then work as a large unit and its success will be judged by CMS against prevailing standards. States a *Forbes* summary: "The providers in an ACO are responsible for management and care of the health plan enrollees and are financially rewarded if the enrollees or patients stay out of the more expensive hospital."[17]

At least, that's the theory.

I belong to an ACO called Northern Maryland Collaborative Care. One day last year I received a letter and email asking me to join and describing the general philosophy of accountable care organizations, something I had read about at length but did not fully understand. Essentially I would be working with a large group of unnamed doctors in my region in an unspecified manner to somehow reduce cost. By joining, I would not relinquish any component of my current relationship with Medicare; my payments would not change for seeing patients, the rules would not change, and the entire care structure would remain intact. According to the provider handbook, ACOs could be composed of professionals in a group practice, networks of individual practices, hospital-professional partnerships, or hospitals that employ professionals, as long as the named group cares for at least five thousand Medicare enrollees and follows a basic organizational structure that the handbook elucidates. In addition, the handbook states that if any of my patients sign up, they too would not lose any of their current benefits or be subject to any new restrictions. States the handbook: "Simply put, there is no change to Medicare benefits whether a patient uses a physician participating in the ACO or not." Patients would be contacted by care coordinators if they did join, both to conduct an initial health assessment and to identify high-risk patients who may need additional services, especially after being in the hospital. The primary goal is to avert future hospitalizations.[18] Not sure what my role in this ill-defined group may be, but assured that I would not be penalized for joining, I signed up.

Since I joined, and have had many (positive) interactions with the ACO representatives, I now have a better understanding of the ACO's mission and its limitations. Most fundamentally, ACOs try to cut health-care costs of its patient base when compared to a benchmark, which is typically the annual cost incurred for the same patient base averaged over the past three years. If there is savings compared to the benchmark, if the savings exceeds a certain minimum, and if the group has practiced "quality" health care, then some of that savings is shared among the ACO and its members. Essentially my ACO carries out two functions to achieve the primary objective of saving money. First, it helps us identify patients who are at high risk for hospitalization and overutilization of medical resources. ACO teams provide care coordination to help such patients stay healthy and navigate the health-care landscape. Second, the ACO monitors our adherence to a set of quality indicators, essentially replacing PQRS with other measures of "quality" to which we must adhere if we are able to share in the savings. If we have passed Medicare's quality indicators and saved money, then some of that money will trickle down to the ACO after the ACO expenses are paid. As of this writing, our ACO has accrued no savings.

Nationally, ACOs have generated $700 million of savings compared to the benchmarks, which translates into a 1 percent drop in Medicare expenses. Of that savings, $300 million has been distributed back to some of the ACOs, and the rest is kept by Medicare. Approximately half of the country's 220 ACOs have achieved some cost reduction, but only fifty-two qualified for shared savings. Currently none of the ACOs take on any risk, but that will change, and those ACOs that are willing to take on the most risk may also be permitted to change some of Medicare's underlying rules, such as eliminating the three-night-stay rule, having more ability to treat people at home, and even having the ability to use tele-medicine.[19] Only time will tell if these reforms are actually utilized by ACOs. Not surprisingly, the majority of ACOs that qualified for shared savings are from areas of the country where health care is most expensive, and thus the benchmark was very easy to beat. States one article: "ACOs from low spending regions argue that the formula used to calculate spending benchmarks inappropriately rewards prior poor performance." This is likely why my ACO failed to achieve shared savings, since our prior performance was actually quite good. In fact, only one out of sixteen ACOs in better performing regions achieved shared savings.[20] Many doctors worry about whether savings can be sustained once benchmarks improve in all groups (since essentially every few years an ACO will have to compete against its own prior performance), and whether ACOs will have to risk losing money once the rules change. Of course, in a small ACO, poor performance by only a few doctor groups in the ACO can cost the entire ACO its ability to save money, something that every other doctor in the ACO cannot control. Also, many observers believe that the early savings generated by ACOs are due to their ability to identify the most onerous problems in the most poor performing areas of the country, and that there will not be continued savings generated once this low-lying fruit is fixed, especially if ACOs do not allow for substantive alterations of Medicare's rules and payment schedules.

At an AMDA conference about which I previously wrote several talks about ACOs only further confused me, although I did learn that they would become required for all doctors in several years.[21] A *Washington Post* article in July 2013 confirmed that as the program is being phased in, doctors will start to be penalized for poor "quality" performance. A doctor's quality grade will be based on adherence to the very clinical guidelines we have already discussed, and by how much each ACO's average patient costs the system.[22] According to a *JAMA* study, the thirty-three quality measures being employed by ACOs do not have a clear correlation to a population's health. In fact, the study concludes that the overall ACO structure lacks the incentives and structure to really improve a population's overall health as it does not focus on long-term determinants of outcome for the elderly.[23] The quality indicators to which we are required to adhere—including placing elderly people with certain cardiac conditions on a preset group of medicines despite their inability to tolerate such drugs, and keeping all of our elderly patients' blood pressures below 120, which clearly can be detrimental to this group—do not allow us to care for our patients as individuals, while incenting us to check boxes and not discuss issues with our patients.

For me in particular, an ironic twist is built into the ACO grading system. Since we are judged by how often our patients are hospitalized, and since so many of my patients are in assisted-living facilities, which in our county are hot spots of hospitalization, I may emerge as one of the most egregious hospitalizers in the entire ACO. By not altering the rules of long-term care, and by not making assisted-living facilities partners in the

ACO process, health-care reformers have provided absolutely no incentive for those facilities to avert hospitalization, something that the current Medicare and regulatory system both encourages and finances. Also, there is nothing built into the ACO model that incentivizes patients and families to stay out of the hospital. Thus, my patient population will likely continue to flock to the hospital, something that is completely out of my control but is now something for which I will be held accountable. I suppose that is why this is considered accountable care!

By not changing the infrastructure of health-care delivery and by not altering how doctors are paid, ACOs are trying to accomplish what HMOs could not without having any power to alter the behavior of those who benefit from a more specialized and aggressive health-care model. As one observer concludes, the current model "works against the very design of the program. The inequities of the fee-for-service system, which rewards proceduralists and specialists at the expense of cognitive specialties and primary care, remain embedded in the payment system."[24] In the old HMO model, especially the one I so appreciated at the retirement community where I worked, primary-care doctors had a central role in medical decision making, absurd concepts like the three-day rule were eliminated, home health was better financed and made more creative, and patients had some skin in the game since they received more services if the Medicare Advantage Plan saved money. None of this is true in ACOs. One study done at the inception of the ACO model explains that "primary care physicians have little direct leverage over other providers in the care continuum, and under the largely fee-for-service payment system it is unlikely other providers will respond to reductions in the number of referrals or admissions by allowing their incomes to fall." Also, the success of ACOs is limited by the concern that "hospitals and specialists would garner a disproportionate share of any savings."[25]

In fact, I do not truly understand how the ACO is going to help me save the system money and provide better care to my patients. Other than charting numbers, and offering care-coordination nurses, the ACO has done nothing to alter the scope of my practice. I do not coordinate care with other doctors; I do not even know which other doctors are in my ACO. I still have no tools to treat people at home rather than in the hospital, and patients continue to be incentivized financially to be hospitalized when they are very ill. I have no extra time to converse with my patients, and much of my patient encounter continues to be (perhaps even more so) focused on typing notes in my EMR and checking off quality measures. In fact, discussions with patients may actually be counterproductive, especially if those discussions lead patients to not be immunized or screened for cancer, or to stop certain medicines for blood pressure or heart disease because those medicines are making them sick, all of which are required so that I can prove I practice quality medicine.

Although the ACO model relies on care coordination by nurses and social workers to nudge patients down a more sensible clinical path away from the hospital, that idea has proven to be more expensive and complicated than anticipated, especially given the lack of primary-care doctors who have time to help facilitate the process.[26] An early ACO medical-home project, in which funds were directed to primary-care doctors and community groups to improve care of those with chronic illness, saved the system $168 per patient, at a cost of $240 per patient, without any perceived improvement in health outcome.[27] Another demonstration project, the Pioneer ACO, did somewhat better, cutting expenses by 4 percent in the first year, but those cuts started diminishing in the second year, and some experts warn that the potential benefit of ACOs may be limited to a brief duration of time that is not sustainable.[28] While care coordination is a worthy and potentially beneficial goal, it cannot by itself dam the flow of aggressive treatment that dominates our health-care-delivery system. To advise patients to stay out of the hospital, but then have nothing else to offer them in the way of home and palliative care, prevents care coordinators from truly making a dent in Medicare's flawed payment model. ACOs represent a noble and thoughtful idea, but one without any teeth in the landscape of geriatric health-care delivery.

Bundled Payment System

Another potentially promising innovation is that of bundled payments, a concept driven by hospitals that is designed to reduce the cost of post-hospital care and curtail the high rate of hospital readmissions from long-term-care facilities. It is due to be fully enacted in 2019. Bundled payment systems are a rendition of diagnosis-related groups (DRGs) that Medicare codified in 1982 and that have shaped hospital spending ever since. Under DRGs hospitals are paid a certain bundled fee for each diagnosis with which a patient presents, despite how long a patient stays in the hospital for that diagnosis. Medicare has devised 467 diagnosis groups for which it will always pay a set fee.[29] Bundled payments take this concept a step further. Now hospitals will be paid a set fee for both the acute hospital stay *and* all services that are required thirty days after the hospital stay, including rehabilitation stints, home health, and even rehospitalization. The goal of bundling patients is to encourage hospitals to identify patients who are at high risk of being readmitted to the hospital and to manage them better to avoid readmissions. Currently it is believed that up to 20 percent of patients are readmitted to the hospital within thirty days of discharge, a high cost to the system. Bundling will incentivize hospitals to cut down this number.[30] I will note that in my patient population, readmissions constitute a very small percentage of overall admissions, and certainly are nowhere near the 20 percent that is cited. Of the large number of hospital admissions that occurred in my long-term patients during the six-week period I was tracking those numbers (see chapter 5), only one or two were readmissions. Thus in my world, bundled payment would impact a tiny proportion of total hospitalizations.

In fact, in a perverse way, bundled payments may *encourage* hospitalization. Without hospitalizing patients in the first place, hospitals and their contracted agents (physicians, home-health services, nursing homes, etc.) will never see the profits that bundled care promises. And after their thirty-day posthospital stint, it certainly makes financial sense to hospitalize patients again to initiate another bundle. As one study stated, "In an effort to maintain income levels that are necessary to cover fixed costs, providers may change their behaviors to increase the volume of episodes." "Episodes" here refers to hospitalizations.[31] Bundling payments could also be medically deleterious to patients by denying them certain facets of care (in an effort to cut cost) in the posthospital period. In fact, the real incentive is not to help the patient have better long-term outcomes, but rather to help them do well enough in the thirty-day posthospital period so that they stay out of the hospital for that brief stretch of time. One study states that bundling "in some instances could produce unintended consequences that would contribute to avoidable poor outcomes" among the vulnerable elders,[32] especially when it comes to their long-term outcomes.

Bundling does not erase many of the ingredients that trigger hospitalization in the first place. The three-day rule will still exist, meaning that facilities and patients both will profit if a patient stays in the hospital for three nights. Also, the current liability and regulatory environment will not be repaired, both of which encourage hospitalization and aggressive care. Virtually every factor we discussed that drives the excessive use of hospitalization among the frail elderly will be left intact outside of the thirty-day window. As with ACOs, bundling payments does not alter the basic skeleton of our health-care-delivery system that pushes patients to embrace specialization and hospitalization. I am also skeptical of any reform effort that is controlled by the hospital itself. That seems to be a very backward method of reducing hospitalization!

The Independent Payment Advisory Board (IPAB)

One stipulation of the ACA is the initiation of a payment advisory board that will help guide Medicare policy and recommend pay scales for physicians. The IPAB, which is very controversial among politicians, is a fifteen-member independent panel appointed by the president and confirmed by the Senate. The members are supposed to be nationally recognized experts in health finance, payment, economics, and actuarial science. There is no stipulation that any doctors sit on the board, and certainly no expectation that practicing doctors like me would even be invited. The board would be able to instigate changes in Medicare with limited congressional input.[33]

A war of words has been waged on the Internet regarding the potential impact of the IPAB. Howard Dean, a physician, former governor, and past chairman of the Democratic National Committee, states that similar rate-setting programs have a forty-year track record of failure. Such a board will not cut costs, he contends. He also points to a perceived flaw of the board, that a top-down approach to health-care reform will not be well accepted: "patients and physicians get aggravated because bureaucrats . . . are making medical decisions without knowing the patient."[34] Peter Orszag, who helped to create the IPAB, counters that the board is necessary to guide Medicare into a new era. The board, he states, will be "tweaking our evolving payment system in response to incoming data and experience."[35] Currently legislation is being regularly introduced to eliminate the board entirely, even though it is not even projected to be organized until 2023.[36] Until then, the old formulas will remain intact, meaning that reimbursement will inevitably favor specialists and procedures.

From all we know about Medicare reform and what needs to be accomplished, it is hard to imagine that a group of politically appointed "experts" who have no firsthand experience with the practice of medicine will be able to transcend their parochial perceptions and create a sensible health-care-delivery system for seniors. Unless practicing primary-care and geriatric physicians (along with their patients) are involved in crafting reform, the result is likely to be a complicated, formulaic strategy that misses the point. As I have suggested throughout this book, we in primary care know what is wrong with Medicare and how to save it. We understand why current policy will not be effective, for many of the reasons I have elucidated. And we know what barriers stand in the way. The only problem we have is that no one ever asks us.

Chronic Care Management (CCM)

Medicare is now paying primary-care doctors up to $40/month to manage chronic care. This is a novel reform; doctors will now be paid for work they do that transcends office visits. We can talk to patients, meet with families, fill out forms, and discuss issues with nurses for a small fee. The implementation of the plan is onerous, the note we are required to write is very complicated and time-consuming, and patients must agree to be part of the program and accept a small co-pay each time the CCM encounter occurs. We also all fear that the CCM program will generate more audits and possible fines if we do not strictly follow the confusing rules. It is unclear if CCM encounters will reduce costs, improve care, or make any dent in the current Medicare dysfunction.

The Medicare Innovation Center (CMMI)

With a staff of nearly three-hundred employees, and a budget of 10 billion dollars over ten years, the CMMI (Center for Medicare and Medicaid Innovation) is a part of the ACA designed to finance projects initiated in the medical community that will improve quality care and reduce cost. Most recipients of awards are hospitals, insurance companies, states, nursing homes, and some community groups. Such projects are localized experiments that, if successful, can be broadened to impact larger groups of patients, and perhaps alter Medicare itself. Accountable Care Organizations

(ACOs) are one result of the CMMI's efforts. But as with much the CMMI is doing, the actual utility of ACOs is unknown and, at least to many primary care doctors, just another burden placed on our laps without being constructed with the input of practicing physicians and without having any proven benefit.

While experimentation is both necessary and laudable, it is unclear whether the primary recipients of CMMI's dollars are simply more bureaucratic agencies that are out of touch with the realities of Medicare and geriatric medicine. Certainly, as with much of the current reform thrust, primary-care input is either lacking or absent. Also, without making more fundamental changes in the structure of Medicare, all such efforts are merely Band-Aids that will be slapped on a dysfunctional system, thereby assuring their inability to usher in meaningful change. Rather than simply financing pockets of innovation, perhaps the government should determine which broad changes will be most effective. From there, then real experimentation can begin.

Total Payment Revenue Budget Cap

A novel and potentially exciting plan that is gaining a foothold in my state of Maryland involves having the government pay hospitals a global monetary budget every year to provide all health-care services. Under such a system hospitals will be more profitable if they can reduce their hospital costs, cut down admissions, and maintain a healthy patient population. Presumably hospitals would work with community organizers, doctors, and nursing homes to keep patients out of the hospital by improving outcomes and health prevention. If they provide global care cheaper than their historical revenue norms, they profit. If not, they may lose money. Some worry that such a plan will induce hospitals to turn away patients who need hospitalization and to curtail important services. Others believe that hospitals will have no control over admissions and may be put in a precarious financial position.[37]

Ideally, a capitated hospital will be the perfect engine to drive an effective home-care model. Bypassing Medicare, hospitals can pay doctors, long-term-care facilities and home-health agencies directly to keep people out of the hospital, no longer having to adhere to the three-day rule. They can pay for short subacute stays, IV treatments, physical therapy, even custodial care; such payments would save them money if they could keep people out of the hospital. But they may still be hampered by long-term-care regulations, by legal liability, and by fear of fraud. It is unclear whether Medicare would even allow such an arrangement to exist. And ultimately hospitals, which would have total control over the entire process, may resort to business as usual, finding other ways to cut costs.

In reality, the most daunting fear that some of us have about such a plan is the centrality of the hospital in scripting it. Likely hospitals will attempt to maximize their own profits by deflecting costs elsewhere in the system, perhaps to outpatient sites that they will own, perhaps to other facilities that perform similar roles such as subacute centers, perhaps to doctors who will have to care for sicker patients without appropriate resources. While this may in itself spur creative ways to care for patients outside the dangerous and expensive hospital walls, it may also simply shift care to other locations no less dangerous and much less sustainable. Also, it must be realized that under current Medicare rules, patients make their own decisions as to whether they choose to utilize the hospital for care, and unless they are incented to stay out of the hospital, there is no advantage for patients to cooperate with the hospitals' goals. Doctors, too, have no incentive to be part of such a plan unless the hospitals buy their practices and make them salaried employees, something that has accentuated under this model,[38] or unless somehow doctors are paid and given adequate resources to keep patients out of the hospital. In fact, the end result may be that hospitals will control such a large portion of the entire health-care-delivery landscape that it is up to them whether successful Medicare reform can be enacted. Whether that is a good recipe for better geriatric care at lower cost has yet to be determined; hospitals do not have a good track record of providing sensible geriatric care. But the capitation may be enough of an incentive to nudge them in the right direction.

Trying a Different Approach

My experiences with patient care, and ongoing consultation with very experienced colleagues, have led me down a different road than the one current reform efforts are sending us. While I laud both CMS and the ACA for working to fix a difficult problem, and even for implementing many

novel and potentially beneficial solutions, I cannot imagine that these reforms will be successful without a central role for primary-care doctors
and without a more profound alteration of the current payment and education system. Thus I propose another way forward.

The crux of my reform ideas center on the basic premise of this book:
that aggressive care is not good for older patients, but that Medicare and
other players in our health-care-delivery network are pushing reluctant
patients down that dangerous and expensive path. My script does not assume that incentivizing or punishing doctors and hospitals and even drug
companies will fix the system. And rather than institute an HMO style
of care that shackles patients with unpopular restrictions, true Medicare
reform should help and encourage patients to pursue the sensible and less
expensive options they typically seek. The vast majority of our elderly
want to be treated at home and do not desire aggressive care when it is
futile. Our current system, even with the proposed reforms that are being
implemented, encourages patients to pursue care that most of them do not
actually want. The goal of reform, then, is to provide an alternative health-
care-delivery structure that puts power in the hands of well-informed patients who can control the course of their care. The three basic ingredients
of any successful reforms are as follows:

- **Create a system that is medically sound.** Our health-care system should
  promote care that is individualized, based on patient preference, and
  provides medical interventions that have been shown to be beneficial to
  the specific individuals who are being treated.
- **Create a system that is cost effective.** Any reforms must be able to pay
  for themselves and even reduce system costs. For Medicare to survive
  into the future, it must become financially viable.
- **Create a system that patients want.** Ultimately, patient satisfaction is
  crucial to any successful health-care system. Each patient has unique
  needs and wants, and thus reforms must not be rigid, and ultimately
  should give patients choices. Also, reforms should enhance the doctor-
  patient relationship and the office-visit experience.

Given the history of reform efforts in this country, and the political di-
visiveness that will inevitably impact any calls for change in an entrenched
Medicare structure, it is important that reforms be pragmatic and palatable

to various organizations and perspectives. For instance, if reforms are seen as rationing care, restricting care, putting too much power in the hands of bureaucrats, costing too much, or threatening large organizations such as hospitals or insurance companies, then such reform will never survive its journey through Congress. We all have very specific goals in reforming Medicare, but in this case compromise is crucial. Again, we in primary care understand the nuts and bolts of health-care provision, and we can help steer reform efforts away from ideological constructs and more toward pragmatic fixes.

Rather than script a specific platform for change, I will relay a few basic strategies that can enable us to move toward the more universal goals of improved health care at lower cost and with greater patient satisfaction. These ideas flow from the pages of my book, from my experiences as a primary-care doctor, and from the medical literature. They are certainly not complete or absolute. But they are a start.

Shared Decision Making: Building True Quality into the System

Knowledge is power, but only when that knowledge is accurate and when it is part of a facile conversation between doctor and patient. If this book demonstrates anything, it is that true quality care is not achieved by over-testing, overtreating, and overmedicating people; often less is more when it comes to achieving optimal medical outcomes, especially as people age. Real health-care reform need not rely on rationing to achieve its goals. Rather, once patients understand that the aggressive path—which society has pounded into them as being most thorough and most medically sound—can actually be dangerous and medically impotent, then many of them will chose to purse interventions that are actually more beneficial to them and less costly to the system. MRIs for back pain, screening stress tests, multiple specialist visits, hospitalizations, excessive medication use, even dialysis can be shown, in many cases, to be less efficacious than often much less expensive alternatives. Ultimately doctors and patients must be able to together reach shared decisions about what constitutes the best medical interventions for each particular patient, rather than rely on insurance-mandated generic templates and quality indicators.

Doctor-patient communication is not only crucial to an effective health-care system, it is also what patients most seek. The Association of American Medical Colleges states that patients rate communication as the most important factor in choosing doctors, more than board certification, level of education, and years of training. But often that communication is skewed, with doctors telling patients what to do based on practice guidelines, and patients simply following their orders. States a 2015 editorial in the *Baltimore Sun:* "Medicine still depends, arguably now more than ever, on the two people in the room having a meaningful exchange of information, and we need to continue to develop and build on this essential relationship."[39]

For shared decision making to be successful, doctors and patients need to have access to accurate health-care information. Currently medical publications, the media, pharmaceutical firms, and many doctors themselves relay medical information in contrived relative-risk formats. Consequently, patients cannot make rational decisions about what constitutes the best course of health care. They are led to think that more testing and more treatment lead to better outcomes because the information on which they are basing their decisions is flawed. When patients and doctors sit in an office to discuss medical options, both should be speaking the same language: that of actual risk-benefit. We must implore the media to present information only in that format, and doctors too should be persuaded to present all information using numbers that make sense and which are individualized for that particular patient. A recent survey suggests that less than 10 percent of patients were given accurate information by their doctors about the harms of overdiagnosis regarding cancer screening.[40] When patients used decision aids and were given comprehensible information about overdiagnosis as part of a conversation on breast-cancer screening, they were more likely to make a decision based on their personal preferences rather than what they were told to do.[41]

In many ways, the very fate of health-care reform hinges on the conversation between doctor and patient. When patients are told what to do in relative terms ("You have atrial fibrillation, so you have to take Coumadin, which will cut your risk of stroke by 50 percent"), they are more likely to dive into aggressive care, believing that to be the only sensible and thorough path to take. Many of my patients who have such a conversation with their cardiologist believe that they have no other choice than to take a blood thinner like Coumadin. But when doctors and patients discuss issues using actual risk and benefits ("People with atrial fibrillation do have about a 6/1,000 decreased risk of disabling stroke if they take Coumadin, but they also have about a 12/1,000 increased risk of serious bleeding as well as other side effects, so we should talk about whether this drug is right for you"), they are more likely to carefully consider medical interventions before blindly accepting them. This will reduce overdiagnosis, overtreatment, and overmedication without having to incentivize doctors to ration care. Many patients will eschew interventions that have small benefit and potential risk, especially when they actually understand what those benefits and risks are.

For shared decision making to be effective, several criteria will have to be met:

- We need to develop a universal decision-making tool to be used by the media, by drug companies, and by doctors and patients when they converse. Several such tools exist now, and many professionals are working to develop new methods that can be universally applied. Such tools should use only actual risk-benefit in assessing interventions, should be easy for patients to comprehend, and should have the capacity to be individualized. Erik Rifkin and I in our book *Interpreting Health Benefits and Risks: A Practical Guide to Facilitate Doctor-Patient Communication* present a theatrical depiction of actual risk and benefit. Using one-thousand-seat theaters, we blacken the number of seats that are impacted by medical interventions, both positive and negative. For instance, in a one-thousand-seat theater looking at Coumadin, six seats will be blackened for disabling stroke prevention, twelve seats will be blackened for significant bleeding, both able to be individualized for each patient (see figure 1).[42] David Newman, on his website www.thennt.com, provides actual risk-benefit numbers for many common conditions, including the impact of Coumadin on afib, which is written in clear prose that can be used by patients and doctors during an office conversation. Harlan Krumholz from Yale has devised a concept called PSR (percentage the same result), which describes what the chance of having the same clinical outcome would be whether a patient pursues an intervention or not. For atrial fibrillation, the PSR would be that there is a 99.4 percent chance of avoiding a disabling stroke whether a patient takes Coumadin

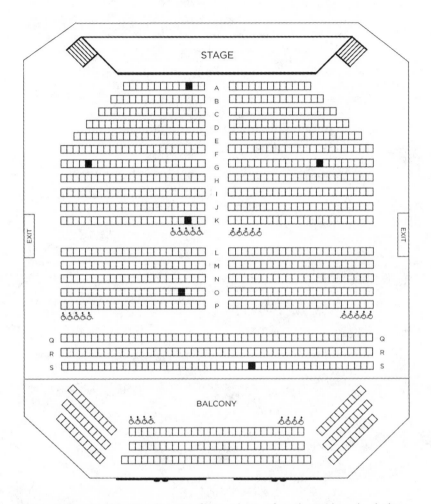

Figure 1. Benefits of anticoagulation in afib. In a theater of one thousand people who have atrial fibrillation deemed at moderate risk of stroke who take Warfarin, approximately six of them will avoid a disabling stroke in a year compared to one thousand people with atrial fibrillation who take aspirin.

or not. Currently the National Physician Alliance and *Consumer Reports* are jointly working on an app that would enable actual data to be obtainable on a smartphone. Regardless of the mechanism, the development of a universal decision-making tool is essential for shared decision making.

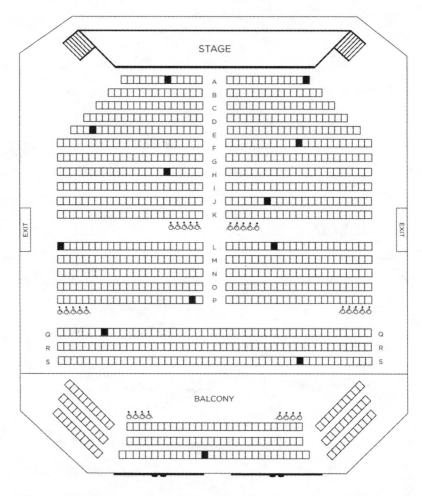

Figure 2. Risk of anticoagulation in afib. In a theater of one thousand people who have atrial fibrillation deemed at moderate risk of stroke who take Warfarin, approximately twelve of them will suffer major bleeds (including bleeds in the brain) compared to one thousand people with atrial fibrillation who take aspirin.

- With a universal decision aid at their disposal, doctors and patients will be able to sit and discuss the benefits and risks of interventions. But for this to occur, doctors will need time to carry out a meaningful conversation. Currently many primary-care practices are so strapped by overhead and time constraints that doctors have only fifteen to twenty minutes to spend with each patient, and much of that time is squandered adhering to and documenting Medicare requirements. Many ideas have floated around about how to increase the amount of time primary-care doctors have to converse with their patients, from having direct primary care (doctors paid per patient and not per visit), to a genuine value-based payment system. Stephen Schimpff's book *Fixing the Primary Care Crisis: Reclaiming the Patient-Doctor Relationship and Returning Health Decisions to You and Your Doctor* has an excellent discussion of the topic with some very viable solutions. A group of working primary-care doctors can help achieve this important objective.

- Finally, for doctors and patients to be able to set an agenda that is patient-centered and to make shared decisions based on actual risk-benefit numbers, then the current quality measures being imposed on us by Medicare will need to be completely rewritten. For reasons well delineated in this book, Medicare's quality indicators do not reflect true geriatric quality and try to stamp often irrelevant templates on what should be individualized decisions. They also frequently encourage more aggressive care that is not always medically sound, which costs more, and which patients do not typically seek. Using the Coumadin example, doctors who simply insist that patients take Coumadin are rewarded by current guidelines, while doctors who discuss the risks and benefits of Coumadin with their patients with the results that some of their patients decide not to take Coumadin will be punished. Perhaps useful quality indicators would simply assess whether doctors have conversations with their patients about specified medical interventions. Regardless, quality indicators should facilitate shared decision making and not stand in the way.

Patient Choice: Building True Value into the System

If knowledge is power, then the capacity to actually use that knowledge in pursuit of quality outcomes is value. It is not enough for doctors and patients to realize that hospitalization is not optimal for many medical conditions, but then be confronted by a medical insurance that will pay only for hospitalization and not any alternatives. Currently Medicare's payment structure drives patients and doctors down a road of aggressive care by financing the most costly services, and not paying for more sensible care that patients may actually prefer. While Medicare pays for MRIs, orthopedic visits, drugs, spinal injections, emergency room visits, and surgery when a patient has back pain, it will not pay for acupuncture and many home devices and treatments that may be more efficacious at a far lower cost, and which patients actually would want. While Medicare pays for endless specialty visits, expensive tests, drug treatments, and ultimately multiple hospitalizations for people with dementia, it will not finance exercise programs, day care, home care, caregiver support groups, and other much less expensive and more useful interventions that so many families seek. A patient who understands the risks and benefits of medical intervention will, when given the choice, often pursue the less interventional option. As we have shown, most elderly want to avoid hospitals, want to die at home, do not want to be on handfuls of medicines, and consider comfort and dignity their primary objectives. Thus incenting doctors to save the system money by somehow keeping their patients away from expensive interventions (what HHS has labeled value) cannot work unless their patients are actually capable of taking a less aggressive route, such as by getting care at home for pneumonia instead of being hospitalized because of Medicare's payment system, something not addressed by Medicare or any current reforms being proposed. If patients are given genuine choices, then it is very likely that they will take a road that makes medical sense, and that road is far less expensive and of much higher value than the one we are on now.

One salient example of Medicare's perverse payment system preventing true patient choice has to do with the three-day rule. As we have discussed, patients who are hospitalized for three nights receive ample benefits: they not only obtain twenty-four-hour care in hospital, receive free intravenous medicines and fluids when necessary, and have medical equipment and oxygen given to them without the need for paperwork, but they are also entitled to one hundred days of inpatient rehabilitation subsequent to their hospital stay, benefits not available to patients treated at home. Doctors who send patients to the hospital have it easier too; it is far more time-consuming and costly for doctors to try to treat patients at home, and the legal system currently puts fear in the minds of doctors who do not hospitalize their ill patients. We know that home care for elderly patients has been shown to be medically superior to hospital care in many cases, is far less expensive, and is what the majority of patients want. In a medical system that seeks true value, physicians and patients should be able to make the decision for home care, and to institute home care easily and without financial penalty. The three-day rule must die, and the incentives pushing people into the hospital must be altered, for this to occur. Give patients a choice, and they will pick value much of the time. It really is that simple.

Recently Congress instituted a new "doc fix" that reversed a several-decade rule that sought to save Medicare money by cutting physician re-imbursement. As part of the new plan, patients can no longer rely on their secondary insurance to pay for their deductible, and there is talk too that perhaps if patients are forced to pay for some of their care, rather than relying on secondary insurances to pay everything that Medicare does not, then they will have more skin in the game, and thus be less likely to pursue aggressive tests and procedures that cost a lot and are not necessarily effective. States the *Washington Post* in its editorial about the doc fix: "Economic theory suggests that patients will use medical services excessively when they face little or no out-of-pocket cost; numerous studies of Medigap [another name for secondary insurance] have concluded that this is indeed what happens. The result is more use of services and higher costs for everyone. Therefore, Medicare reformers on both sides of the aisle have argued that limitations on Medigap could do a lot to bend the curve of rising health-care costs."[43] Such a system would essentially add co-pays for every service; all patients in Medicare would pay a part of every service, from seeing their doctor to getting an MRI. Perhaps creative co-pays will incent patients to move down a more sensible path of health care, and to give them pause before rushing into very expensive tests, procedures, and hospital stays. But until Medicare actually alters its payment structure such restrictions do not meaningfully allow choice within the landscape of health-care provision. Rather, they punish patients for pursuing the only course that is given to them by Medicare. Again, value does not come from restriction of care, it derives from expansion of care: do not tell patients what they cannot do, but give them more options about what they can do.

As a caveat to patient choice, it is important to say a word about malpractice. As we have discussed, the fear of malpractice often persuades doctors to recommend the most aggressive and invasive care for their patients. Currently too many doctors believe that they will be better protected from litigation by ordering more tests, sending people to more specialists, and hospitalizing people more often, despite what a patient actually wants. Fixing the malpractice system is a crucial prerequisite for a genuine patient-focused value-laden health-care delivery system. Congress took a small step in this direction when it passed legislation on the doc fix. Doctors can no longer be sued for adhering to quality guidelines or Medicare's incentives and programs.[44] More needs to be done, though, to create a system that provides patients some protection from medical errors, while not subjecting doctors to what are often frivolous suits.

Palliative Care: Building Genuine Patient Satisfaction into the System

We have talked about palliative care a great deal in this book. Put simply, with a palliative approach we treat symptoms and help people feel better rather than chase numbers, screen for problems, or try to fix the incurable. Palliative care flows from shared decision making; it presumes that patients will orchestrate much of their own care by focusing on what matters most to them. Palliative care is not no care. Doctors still perform tests and discuss issues of treatment and screening with their patients. But the focus of care is to help patients live a better life.

In the elderly, and in people with chronic disease, studies have suggested that a palliative approach not only leads to better patient satisfaction and improved quality of life, but can also lead to a longer life. Overtreating blood pressure, ordering multiple screening tests, exposing a patient to thorough cardiac testing and treatment, and using statins and Coumadin (much of which is mandated by quality indicators) have never been shown to lead to higher quality of life in the elderly or, in many cases, a prolongation of life. In fact, just the opposite is often true, as we have shown in this book and which has been well documented. More significantly, many patients prefer to eschew aggressive care, and they are looking for an alternative approach. Palliative care is what so many elderly truly seek. And in addition to improving outcome, it is far less expensive than the slate of medical options Medicare offers its beneficiaries.

In this country, we often associate palliative care with hospice. As we have discussed, hospice offers people expansive services when they are at the end of life, at a cost to Medicare of $5,000 or more every month. But hospice is restricted only to people who are deemed likely to die within six months. In the frail elderly, especially people with dementia living in nursing homes, hospice is often initiated as the only feasible way of keeping people out of the hospital, but many of those people live longer than six months. A study published in 2015 showed that while hospice does reduce hospitalization in nursing-home patients, it actually costs Medicare more than it saves, primarily because so many residents enroll and they do not immediately die.[45] Remember the hospice effect: often the elderly live longer when we stop testing them and overwhelming them with pills. If you look at hospice through the lens of cost-cutting, hospice is a double-edged sword. It is used for people who are at the end of life, but by offering them quality palliative care, they end up living longer, thus costing the system more money—though not as much as they would spend on aggressive, thorough care.

The lessons of hospice as it is currently constructed under Medicare are complex. First, the frail elderly and people with chronic disease actually benefit from palliative care. They live better and happier, and can live longer. Second, many of the elderly seek palliative care, especially those in long-term care. As we have discussed, the vast majority of elderly do not want to die in a hospital or even a nursing home; they want to be kept comfortable. And yet, unless they are eligible for hospice, they often have no option other than the aggressive route. Third, palliative care reduces expensive and often cruel hospitalization. It is only more expensive than traditional care because current hospice fees are very high. So that raises the question: Can Medicare offer palliative care more broadly to the elderly at a lower cost?

Diane Meier, a pioneer of palliative care who runs an innovative hospital-based palliative care program at Mount Sinai in New York, wrote an excellent summary of palliative care in the *Milbank Quarterly*.[46] She defines palliative care's focus as "achieving the best-possible quality of life for patients and their family caregivers, based on patient and family needs and goals and independent of prognosis." She shows that palliative-care teams—composed of physicians, nurses, social workers, and others—that treat the sickest people with chronic disease increase quality and reduce cost fairly consistently, while often prolonging life. Patients enrolled in palliative care are more likely to remain in their own homes, and less likely to be hospitalized or subjected to overtreatment and overtesting. Palliative care is also less expensive than traditional care. But palliative teams are difficult to find, and Medicare will not reimburse their services. While the ACA allows alternative programs such as ACOs to use palliative teams in their intervention, there is no stipulation about how they will be financed.

Really, though, palliative care need not be a difficult provision for Medicare to institute. Many older people with dementia want very simple services: home-health aides, medical day care, medical care at home, exercise programs, care coordination, even diapers. They do not want specialist and emergency-room visits when they are sick, and prefer to be on fewer medicines and to be tested less. So why can't Medicare offer patients a palliative-care option, where they will relinquish some of their acute-care benefits (perhaps by charging them a sizable deductible for all but primary care and basic medical services), but provide some funding for palliative teams, home-health aides, long-term-care fees, medical day care, extensive home health, and basic medical needs?

For such an option to work in long-term care, the current regulatory environment will need to be restructured. Instead of focusing on numbers, tests, falls, and poor outcomes, regulations should emphasize comfort and dignity. While certain regulations need to maintain as their primary objective the safety of long-term-care residents, the pursuit of medical minutiae that they now endorse is not in concert with a palliative approach to care. Perhaps, too, if in a palliative program patients are given some funds to pay for custodial care, then innovative home-care services can be created that efficiently and effectively allow families to keep their loved ones at home, thus mitigating the need for long-term care in many cases. In either venue, palliative care can deliver quality and value at low cost and with high patient satisfaction.

Increase the Number of Primary-Care Doctors

No reform effort can survive with a primary-care shortage and an overabundance of specialists. We have discussed the benefits of a primary-care-centered health-care system for the elderly in terms of being cost-efficient and improving outcome. Many of the current reforms being instituted by the ACA and Medicare, as well as the reforms other doctors and I have proposed, rely on a robust primary-care presence. A 2015 article concluded that doctors who are more comprehensive in their approach save the system money and lead to a lower hospital rate.[47] To those of us in the field, that is a fact that needs no study. The question is not whether primary care should drive health-care reform. The real question is how to train enough primary-care doctors to enable reform to succeed.

Unfortunately, primary-care doctors are among the most dissatisfied in the country, and few new doctors are entering the field. The Affordable Care Act and novel reforms being heralded by Medicare promised a great deal to those of us in primary care. All the experts touted primary-care doctors as the key to successful health-care reform. Even our president discussed primary care in only the most glowing light. But then reality set in. More paperwork, more regulations, new mandatory programs that are time-consuming and expensive, the threat of government audits with potentially large fines—all of this struck us hard in primary care, and all had been engineered by "experts" in the name of reform. Doctors dropped out of Medicare, others (concierge doctors) eliminated insurance completely and charged patients a fee. Hospitals started buying small practices that could not otherwise survive. Workloads increased and overhead costs escalated, most of it not related to patient care. Many of us feared for our futures. One doctor who sits high on the ladder of CMS (the Centers for Medicare and Medicaid Services) told me that practices like mine would essentially be extinct in the next five years.

This simmering wave of discontent has kept medical students and residents from considering primary care as a profession, sparking a continued decline and projected shortage in the primary-care field. Two articles by Daniela Drake for the *Daily Beast* in April 2014 highlight what many of us in the trenches have known for a long time.[48] Drake begins in one of the articles: "Doctors are miserable, patients are miserable, and there's no end in sight. It's time to revamp the health-care system from the ground up— starting with primary care." The author contends that health-care delivery has been co-opted by "thought leaders" including academics, consultants, and policy experts, while 82 percent of practicing physicians like me "feel powerless to influence the profession." One primary-care doctor she interviewed, who supports a movement to drop out of insurance completely and simply charge patients a membership fee, states that the system is so broken it cannot be fixed. "I always say you can't polish a turd. That's what most pundits and consultants are trying to do: hence the advent of Accountable Care Organizations (ACOs) and patient centered medical home constructs. These do nothing to address the culture. They simply impose more restrictions, mandates, and parameters on dangerously stretched physicians." This is a sentiment with which many of us who practice medicine absolutely agree.

The author states that nine out of ten doctors discourage others from joining the profession, and that many "doctors feel that America has declared war on physicians—and both physicians and patients are losers." The ACA has codified a system in which primary-care doctors are the workhorses with no power to impact change. They are judged by productivity and patient-satisfaction scores, which have little relevance to quality care. "But the primary care doctor doesn't have the political power to say no to anything—so the 'to do' list continues to lengthen. A stunning and unmanageable number of forms . . . show up on a physician's desk needing to be signed. Reams of lab results, refill requests, emails, and callbacks pop up continually on the computer screen. Calls to plead to insurance companies are peppered throughout the day. Every decision carries with it an implied threat of malpractice litigation. Failing to attend to these things brings prompt disciplining or patient complaint. And mercilessly, all of these tasks have to be done on the exhausted doctor's personal time." In my experience, what I love about practicing medicine—spending time with my patients—often takes a backseat to the meaningless busywork we are told to complete, much of it driven by the ACA and Medicare's reforms. Concludes the article: "To be sure many people with good intentions are working toward solving the healthcare crisis. But the answers they've come up with are driving up costs and driving out doctors."

The first and most salient barrier to students entering primary-care fields is the salary discrepancy between primary-care doctors and specialists. We have discussed this in detail, and nothing in the ACA or on the docket of Medicare reform has meaningfully altered that reality. While the purveyors of change suggest that shared savings—the money primary-care doctors will be able to obtain by increasing the quality and value of their care—may help narrow the salary gap, nothing of the sort has yet

occurred. If anything, reforms have just piled more work and greater regulatory burdens on primary-care doctors, making the field even less palatable. A small committee in the AMA still determines salaries, and even
if that is transferred to another small group that has been designated by
the ACA, there is nothing being proposed that will remedy this problem.
Something substantive must be done in this regard if we hope to convince
students to enter primary care.

The nature of premedical and medical education also dissuades students from pursuing primary care. The premed curriculum, largely unchanged from when Abraham Flexner proposed it in 1910, emphasizes
rote memorization of certain areas of science—primarily chemistry, phys-
ics, and biology—that "weeds out" many students who want to enter the
medical field as physicians. Many people like me believe that the premed
requirements do not assess for the important attributes of critical thinking and compassion, and thus many who become doctors lack those skills,
which of course are essential to the pursuit of primary care. Also, the premed years are ones of "aggressive competition for grades that conflicts
with the precepts of medical professionalism: academic and intellectual
rigor, creative thinking, collaboration, and social conscience." A program
at Mount Sinai Medical School accepts a large group of students who do
not fulfill the premed requirements or take the Medical College Admission Test (MCAT), and they perform just as well in medical school as
more traditional students. But even they do not pursue primary-care
fields in large numbers,[49] likely because of the inherent financial and logistical problems primary-care doctors face, as well as the structure of
medical school itself.

As we discussed, medical-school students have very little exposure to
primary care and are taught mostly by specialists, researchers, and academics. Most gravitate to specialty fields, with the promise of more money
and more prestige. Interestingly, Medicare itself can change that reality
very easily. Currently Medicare subsidizes residency medical-training
programs that determine in which field of medicine doctors can achieve
certification. The average cost per student per year paid by Medicare to
hospitals for such training is $112,641, or $10 billion dollars overall a year.[50]
Given the scope of that investment, Medicare should have some discre-
tion as to who can get trained in which fields. If we do have a primary-
care crisis, Medicare can simply increase its funding to primary-care

fields, while reducing funded slots in specialty fields. In 1997 Congress froze funding for residencies because of escalating costs, and thus almost 90 percent of US medical school deans are concerned that there will not be enough training slots available for their graduates.[51] Perhaps by increasing the ratio of primary care to specialty funded slots, Medicare can provide adequate training slots without having to invest more money into a bloated system.

Medical school debt is another contributor to career choice. Graduating with $200,000 debt does not permit most medical students the luxury of following a path of primary care. Some researchers have contemplated cutting medical school by a year in an effort to save money without sacrificing quality. One study concluded that "there is substantial waste in the education and training of US physicians. Years of training have been added without evidence that they enhance clinical skills or quality of care. This waste adds to the financial burdens of young physicians and increases health care costs."[52]

Interestingly, a 2014 *Washington Post* article about this topic talks about eliminating the fourth year of medical school, which in my opinion is a very crucial year educationally. The article's author interviewed medical-school administrators who suggested that any curtailment would necessarily involve the fourth year, with some claiming that a one-year cut "has been tried before, and it was a miserable failure."[53] But in reality, a revamping and trimming of the two preclinical years (the first two years of most medical schools), including moving at least one of those years to becoming part of the undergraduate premed curriculum, would easily allow medical schools to impart a quality education in three years. With reduction in medical school cost, debt will be a less persuasive factor in career decisions, and this is something that has to be considered more sensibly by reformers. Further, a plan to provide additional debt relief to primary-care doctors will push more students in that direction. Such an investment would produce large dividends if it does increase our primary-care supply. And without more primary-care doctors, Medicare reform cannot succeed.

Ultimately, a primary-care-driven health-care-delivery system that is patient centered and multidisciplinary, relies on shared decision making using actual risk-benefit analysis, offers doctors and patients options for care that are palliative and home-based, and acknowledges the dangers of overtesting and overtreating will be possible only when Medicare becomes an instrument of positive change. Currently, that is not the case. In actuality, Medicare can accomplish this fairly simply by shifting its focus. Medicare can start by eliminating or changing its quality indicators, giving doctors more time to care for their patients, providing doctors and patients with reasonable tools to allow them to be treated at home and in a palliative way, and increasing the number of primary-care doctors.

Many doctors and medical thinkers have determined that Medicare is simply too politically driven and too beholden to special interests to surmount its parochial models of reform. Some suggest that doctors leave all insurance behind and simply charge retainer fees to their patients. If Medicare cuts its costs to allow for its recipients to purchase direct primary care, they argue, then we can construct a primary-care-driven health-care system with the features I have described above. Others suggest that Medicare Advantage Plans may offer more creative ways to spend Medicare dollars outside of the strict rules, regulations, and payment structure that Medicare has imprinted on health-care delivery. Such Medicare HMOs, when primary care based, have shown some success, and their numbers are growing.

Ultimately, though, our goal should not be to discard Medicare, to rely on the private sector, or to give elderly patients vouchers through which they can purchase health insurance, as some have suggested. Medicare has dramatically improved the health care of seniors in this country, and it can continue to pursue that mission. What it will require is more sensible reform. The gap between superb cost-effective care and the bloated system we now live under is not large. But to bridge the gap, it is time we stop relying on "experts" who know nothing of the system they have been asked to shape. Instead, primary-care doctors, who know how to deliver quality care, and their patients should be the architects of change. To start that process, our seniors and their doctors must be given accurate information about what constitutes truly thorough care, and Medicare is poised to be the instrument to finance that care.

Society has defined thorough care as a search for perpetual life by overtreating, overtesting, and engaging in a quixotic quest for the unachievable through specialization and hospitalization. We know that such a definition of thorough is actually counterproductive, and that aggressive care can lead to great harm at significant financial and physical cost. It is also not what most patients and their families actually want. Medicare has encouraged that leap into "thorough" health care through its payment structure and clinical guidelines. But Medicare can and should be the instrument to help us obtain better care for our elders, not the high-cost specialized care that it is financing currently. To those who seek to age gracefully, Medicare can be there in perpetuity to guide us along the way, as long as reform is carried out more sensibly. The first philosophical barrier to address is redefining what thorough care really is for the elderly. We will end the book on that note.

Afterword

REDEFINING THOROUGH

Our society must make it right and possible for old people not to fear the
young or be deserted by them, for the test of a civilization is the way it cares
for its helpless members.

PEARL BUCK, Nobel Prize–winning novelist

Today I saw a patient who looked great. Almost eighty, in a retirement
community, Mrs. W. had come to a certain peace in her life. She had been
very anxious, struggling with pain everywhere, worsening balance, high
blood pressure and high sugar, fatigue, and depression. She saw doctors
and specialists with great regularity, flooded her body with medicines and
tests, and was always looking for a fix. She could not leave her apartment,
and was losing weight. Now all that had improved and she glowed.

"I am fighting the good fight," she told me. "And I am winning."

The good fight had changed its focus over the past few months for Mrs.
W. Until recently she attempted through various devices and doctor visits
to eliminate her pain, to fix her balance and find out why she was so shaky,
to worry about her blood pressure and sugars that she checked incessantly,
to wonder what had become of her now that she had been forced to exist
in a retirement community with so many old people. But at some point an
epiphany overcame her thoughts. Now the good fight meant that she was

going to persevere despite all the problems that gnawed at her. She stopped all but a couple of pills, and her sugars and pressure actually improved. She walked with a walker and had become more social. Now she taught a class on spirituality in her retirement community, helping others to come to peace with themselves.

"I no longer ask why," she told me. "I just move on and do what I can. And I am trying to help others do the same. By helping them, I'm helping myself."

Mrs. W. had come to a point in her life where she stopped trying to cure her aging. She in fact started to redefine "thorough." She no longer adhered to the accepted dogma that with aggressive posturing she could defeat the many ailments and diseases that struck her. She did not chase numbers, ask for more tests, put herself on countless medicines, and seek specialty care. Instead, she accommodated to aging and she thrived. To her, "thorough" no longer implied being tested and treated to death in an effort to achieve something that continued to frustrate and elude her. Now "thorough" meant to work hard in all facets of her life so that she could live and thrive despite her ailments. "Thorough" was not something a doctor or test or drug was going to give to her. It was the mental and physical discipline that was now her responsibility so she could become a healthier and happier person.

Despite all we do not know about medical treatment of the elderly, especially those with memory loss and dementia, we do know that an active lifestyle that emphasizes socialization and exercise can achieve successful improvement in symptoms and quality of life.[1] In my experience, those who look past their ailments and live their lives to the fullest are the ones who age the most successfully and who are the happiest.

One of my favorite patients, ninety-three-year-old Mr. P., was a tiny Italian man who typically came in with his pleasant son for our every-three-months visits. He had a litany of medical problems, most of which were either quiet or of no concern to him, and overall he remained active and healthy, without much to relay to me. He accepted and accommodated to aging very well. His son, too, did not want to look for problems, and often we talked about issues of the day, or other more mundane topics such as the soups they were serving at his retirement community. His son took him on trips frequently, and even became a shuttle driver at the community where his father lived so he could see his father more and help others in his father's shoes.

One day I saw that Mr. P. made an acute visit to see me, and I asked my front staff why he was coming in.

"He wouldn't tell us," the receptionist said to me. "But he said it was urgent that he see you today."

I feared that this man who complained about nothing must have a catastrophic illness; why else would he demand to see me today? But when he arrived in the office, he looked great.

"Hey, doc," he said with his typical smile. "I've got heart disease, diabetes, high blood pressure, I pee too much from a big prostate, and my balance isn't worth a damn. You can write all that stuff in your note and bill Medicare for it and say we talked about it. But let me tell you why I am really here."

I peered at him inquisitively.

"I'm taking a Jewish history class at the community college, which is a great class, but there's a lot of confusing things they talk about for a Catholic like me, and I know you're Jewish, and you like history, so I was wondering if I could run some stuff by you."

That was the urgent visit! And both of us enjoyed it very much.

But after discussing a bit of history, we did talk about him, how he was feeling, what his expectations were for the rest of his life, his exercise regime, his family. I learned more about Mr. P. during that visit than I had in all my previous medical encounters. Never did I put a blood-pressure cuff on his arm, whip out my stethoscope, or suggest checking labs. I did not even dance my hands across the computer keyboard desperately scripting Medicare's requisite note. I merely followed his agenda. For a brief moment I stepped outside the narrow cage into which society and Medicare has shoved me as I care for my patients. Instead I became Mr. P.'s doctor.

Looking back on Mr. P's visit and others that have been similar, I realize that we are defining "thorough" all wrong. To be a thorough doctor is not only about ordering tests and prescribing medicines and checking numbers that we can fix. That is an easy way to satisfy everyone and accomplish nothing. To be really thorough is to hold back from being aggressive. To explain to my patients why certain labs and treatments may not be appropriate despite what they may have read in the *Washington Post* or heard from their neighbor. To have the guts not to listen to their heart with my stethoscope or check their blood pressure. To be thorough is to talk to them about their lives, their futures, their fears, and their limitations and to help them surmount the ravages of aging. That discussion may not always involve an exam or even a medical vocabulary. But it is the most thorough way that we as doctors can interact with and help our elderly patients.

Being thorough is very difficult, because the script tells us and our patients that we are supposed to be checking and looking and measuring. Medicare's formulaic template notes, which doctors must complete at every visit to be compliant with their rules, insist that we assess a specified number of complaints, record a specified amount of measurements, examine a specified amount of their body, and review a specified number of problems. Even Medicare's wellness visit, which was a gift to primary care from CMS because it allows us to spend time with our patients once a year without having to delve into their medical problems, is built with a preordained template of clinical-practice guidelines that we must complete exactly as Medicare states. Unfortunately, that template often does not jibe with my elderly patients' lives or needs, and its questions have no meaning for those who live in long-term care or are too confused to respond. Medicare, and the society that fuels it, has defined "thorough" as being aggressive, and that philosophy is imprinted on every action we are required to take. But that is not what the elderly need and want. And that approach is expensive and ineffective, even if it is the simplest path to take. We as a society, and we as a medical community, must redefine "thorough." That is what will cure Medicare.

The public perception of my profession is a dreary one. The idea of caring for the elderly elicits images of decay, decline, mental collapse, gas, wet diapers, walkers, electric carts, hearing aids, and of course the siren of an ambulance taking yet another old guy to the hospital. All of these images are, of course, correct, and on any given day I am confronted with each of these situations, and I also fill out any number of death certificates, saying good-bye to another of my patients, a victim of the inevitability of aging.

But my job is so much more than that. Its concealed beauty reminds me of my four years of medical school in the North Bronx. When people visited me there they pointed out the congestion, graffiti, and garbage in the street. But being there I became numb to all that. Instead I enjoyed the wonderful food, smells, vitality, and landscape; the best running trails I ever darted on traversed the wilderness of the Bronx. And when I view my job now, I am numb to the overt signs of aging that my patients wear every day and see only beauty. Within each of my patients is a full life that has been lived, a vitality that sadly is often stripped away in their feckless fight to defeat age. Within each of my patients is a story and an enduring spark, and that is what I seek to discover and ferment, rather than merely being a robotic technician who fixes numbers and pushes the false allure of thorough.

The heart and soul of my job emanates from the patients I have the honor to care for and who are so much deeper than the diagnoses and numbers that have come to define them. I have met patients who worked with famous politicians and scientists, and some who shared some quiet fame of their own. I have lived through D-day and Okinawa, have been aboard ships at Midway where explosions caused asbestos snowstorms and the entire crew shit in their pants. I have lived the life of POWs in Germany trading cigarettes for food, and of men on the front line watching as their friends were picked off one by one. Just the other day I met a new patient in his nineties who was on the airfields of Pearl Harbor when it was attacked, when he felt that every Japanese plane that dived down was trying to kill him personally. I have taken care of German women who lived through the bombing of Berlin and witnessed the deaths of most of their family members, and Jews who survived the gas chambers. Even the most dementia-afflicted veterans and war victims I've come to know, the ones who no longer recognize their wife and kids and don't know a spoon from a pen, can recall their military units and battles with clarity and emotion. From teachers to salesmen, to artists and astronauts and victims of racist attacks, my patients are the very embodiments of living history. They relish telling their stories, and in many ways those stories encapsulate who they are and define how they think.

Sadly, it is often only after my patients die that I get to know them. I remember one man with dementia from the nursing home who often climbed into women's beds and spit on the nursing aides. To us, he was quite pathetic. When he died, no one thought much about it. Two days later I picked up a copy of the *Baltimore Sun* and stumbled on a quarter-page

obituary near a picture of a young man smiling brightly, holding a trum-
pet, and surrounded by cheering soldiers. It turns out that this man had
been a key figure in the founding of the USO, and then had gone on to
be a successful corporate leader who helped modernize the army's supply
network. To many people quoted in the obituary, the man was a hero. It
saddened me that I had not known about him before. I cared more about
his blood pressure, his medicines, and his behavior than who he actually
was. Perhaps I could have sparked some of those memories and helped the
man get through what must have been the most painful and demeaning
part of his incredible life.

Throughout my many years of practicing geriatric medicine, I am
most amazed by those patients and families who can look beyond their
problems, who can transcend the overwhelming dogma pounded into
our brains that more is better and that answers and solutions for everything exist if we try hard enough, and who come to peace with their
aging process and learn to live with it by accommodating and persever-
ing. If this book is designed to show anything it is that successful aging
need not be burdened by the constant struggle to defeat the inevitable.
That fight very often leads to disastrous consequences, at a high cost to
the patients and to society. Successful aging is much more rewarding,
and that is what I try so hard to promote at every turn. Unfortunately,
my message that the elderly can best help themselves through physical
and mental discipline is often drowned out by the false hope—trumpeted by pharmaceutical companies, the lay press, specialization, our
medical leaders, and Medicare itself—that there is an answer out there
for everything if you just keep poking yourself enough, taking enough
medicines, and rushing to the hospital when you get too sick. That is my
most daunting enemy, and it is a lethal weed that is choking Medicare's
hope for survival.

It is difficult for most patients and families to view health care
through the lens of common sense. Not when we live in a society that
thrives on excess. There is always a story of someone saved by a procedure or test who is just like Mom. Always a glimmer of hope hanging
just beyond our reach. Always someone who thinks there is an answer
to every problem, or at least there should be. Always a doctor willing to
be the hero.

Therefore, it is up to us to redefine "thorough" and help our patients live better than the dogma allows. I view myself as a guide through the older years, an individual who can help my patients understand, accept, and adjust to the many hazards that barrage us as we age. I try to teach my patients, and their families, to continue living and thriving despite the tide of illness and disability. Rather than medicate people, I try to withdraw medicine. Rather than searching for disease, I try to avoid looking too hard. Rather than aggressively treating ailments such as diabetes and high blood pressure, I try to convince my elderly patients to back off and not worry. To me, the enemies of successful aging are stress and inactivity, and often the quest for immortality through medical thoroughness only accelerates both these demons. I try to retreat from hard-core medical dogma scripted by experts in the form of clinical guidelines, and instead learn to concoct individualized strategies to help my patients maintain their vitality. Sometimes it is difficult for old people and their kids to accept this minimalistic outlook. But medical studies have proven its wisdom, and those of us in the field treat it like gospel based on our ample experience.

Every elderly person lives within a delicate balance between function and disease. Even those who look good externally are standing one insult away from a cascade that may unravel everything. A good doctor knows that. A good doctor is not one who looks for problems, who seeks perfection in numbers, who adds stress to their patients' lives by tossing tests and specialists at them, and who is oblivious to the precarious balance within their patients' bodies. A good doctor is one who knows you well, who holds your hand, and who helps guide you through the medical theater in which you are enjoying the final act. A good doctor has the guts to put on the breaks. When we back off, almost everything improves. Backing off is not giving up. It is the best medicine we have. It is akin to hope. It is truly thorough care.

Medicare does not facilitate successful aging. It does not reward or assist those who take a path of less aggressive care. Often, in fact, it gets in the way. By paying for specialization and hospitalization, for tests and procedures, for the most aggressive care, it sends patients down a road that is traumatic and stressful. By not paying for most home treatments, for nursing aides and phone calls to a doctor, for palliative long-term care and families' ability to keep the elderly at home, Medicare turns its back on quality and dignity.

When I wrote this book, I initially named it after one of my patient's daughters who jokingly anointed herself as "the Boss." The Boss helped me understand that the most thorough patient advocate is not necessarily the one who most bombastically demands to dive into the teeth of a health-care-delivery system that Medicare will gladly finance. Rather, a truly thorough family member, like the Boss, is one who aggressively provides comfort and dignity in someone's final years, and who fights against a system and a society that would have her do otherwise. The Boss was that person, and her thoroughness paid off.

The Boss's mother was my patient for more than a decade. Mrs. Lo was a small, pleasant woman who spoke slowly and repeated herself often. She saw me for visits every three months, typically to discuss her diabetes, some minor aches and pains, and her many stories from Poland, where she was born. Overall Mrs. Lo was very healthy as she entered her nineties, still independent, and not crippled by any serious medical problems. But her mind was slowly deteriorating, and her ability to carry out simple activities of daily living became an increasing burden of which she was never aware but that clearly impacted her life.

I had heard from her daughter sparingly prior to her more pronounced memory loss, but by her mother's late eighties the daughter started to call me often, her voice often tremulous, shooting me a list of Mrs. Lo's most recent sugars, talking about her poor balance, and then asking: "She's going to be OK, right? She's not going to die, right?" The Boss, as she labeled herself because of the fact that she had now put herself in charge of her mom's life, loved her mom as much as anyone ever loved anyone else. She could not imagine life without her.

So, unmarried and without kids, she found a night job and spent her days with her mom. She took her on trips to restaurants and stores, talked about making an excursion to Poland sometime soon, and more than anything kept her mom happy and mobile and independent.

When I first met the Boss she assaulted me with a threatening proclamation: "I want you to know that I am going to do whatever it takes to keep my mother alive, and I expect you to do the same, Doctor." I thought, OK, here's another one of those family members, the ones who treat their parents like little children, drag them from doctor to doctor and test to test, dominate appointments without letting their parents get in a word edge-wise, and ultimately drive their parents into an early and painful grave at great financial and personal expense.

But the Boss was not like that.

Yes, she called me a lot, typically with an alarmist charm about her. But never did she demand anything other than reassurance.

"Mom's diabetes is out of control, Doctor," she said to me, more than just once, reading me a list of sugars that were not very high. "Should we be changing her medicine? Should I be worried? Should we be taking her to an endocrinologist? My sister says these sugars are going to kill her. She is going to be OK, right?"

"Well, those numbers look good to me, but if you want her to go to an endocrinologist, you don't need my permission. Medicare lets you take her to whomever you want whenever you want."

"Doctor, I just want to know that we are doing the right thing and she'll be OK."

"I think she's doing great," I told the Boss.

"Really? She will be OK? Thank you, Doctor. Thank you."

The calls were brief and predictable, and when the Boss called I always called her right back. It took just a minute of time, and once I gave the magic word that all was OK she brought her mom on another walk, or trip, or imaginary adventure in Poland.

And so it went. "Does my mom need a mammogram, Doctor?"

"Not at ninety-two."

"But she'll be all right, right Doctor? She won't die of breast cancer, right?"

"There's probably a higher risk of her getting hit by a car on the way to the test."

"Do you think she'll die of a car accident?"

If I ever suggested a test, or even a specialist appointment as benign as an eye doctor, the Boss bucked. She clearly did not want to put her mother through all of that, even though she asked about it incessantly. Being barraged by a society that believes in excess, the Boss needed constant reassurance from me to do what she knew was right by way of her mother. She needed me to alleviate her stress so she could relieve her mother's. So, from my perspective, everything was OK. Everything would always be OK.

One day the Boss took her mother for a walk in the hall and accidently tripped her mother, who tumbled down and slammed onto her back. Mrs. Lo did not walk again for three months, and the Boss was overcome with guilt. But I continued to deflect the blame (carpets, lighting, poor vision), to help the Boss keep her mom out of a hospital or nursing home (I wrote many letters to her employer to allow her to stay with her mom and arranged some home health, none of which Medicare helped cover), and kept her away from narcotics and specialists and other interventions that might cause her harm. We talked daily on the phone ("She'll be all right, won't she, Doctor? I didn't kill her, did I?"), and I visited her a few times, and eventually Mrs. Lo resumed her car rides and her walks and her dreams about visiting Poland.

One day recently, not long after I left my former job to pursue my own practice, Mrs. Lo had a massive stroke. I talked to the Boss regularly. We discussed hospice, and the Boss agreed to that. "I just don't want her to leave my side," the Boss told me. "I don't want her to have to leave her apartment." I promised her that her mom would stay right there.

I visited Mrs. Lo a few days later. Other relatives were there, and Mrs. Lo was lying in her bed, smiling, mumbling a bit, and staring ahead. The Boss seemed very calm. After my requisite stethoscope to the chest, and after discussing with her what may come next in the dying process, the Boss looked at me and said, "Doctor, thank you so much for coming. Now I know that she'll be OK."

Mrs. Lo died a few days later, in her mid-nineties, in her own bed, her daughter by her side, free of pain or stress, likely thinking about the next car ride and her pending trip to Poland. Medicare paid very little for her care in her final years; she was a bargain for the system. The Boss innately understood the dangers of excess. She went cheap. So many others of my patients and families squander more Medicare dollars in a week than the Boss incurred in a decade. But the Boss considered herself just as thorough and loving as those other patients and families. She wanted the best for her mom. And she delivered on her word.

As a doctor who tries very hard to push my patients off the train of thorough, I know how difficult that is in our current environment. My patients read the papers, watch TV, surf the Internet, talk to friends and medical "experts," are privy to the many "breakthroughs" and "advances" that may help them if they just keep at it. Many buy into the specialized model of care that is so widely revered in this country. The hospital is clearly where most think they need to be if they are very sick, even if aspects of hospitalization frighten them. Many are suspicious of medicines, but want their numbers to look good, are afraid to stop their pills and supplements, believe in ample screening and testing especially if suggested by specialists or other smart people they know (even TV doctors), and cannot shake the idea that cure is possible for nuisance problems and for the inevitable symptoms of aging. Many would rather chase miracles than accommodate, exercise, and work hard at self-improvement.

Even if you incent a doctor like me to do less, which is what so many reforms are attempting, there is no chance of success unless Medicare changes its rules and payments that currently push my patients down a road of aggressive care that even the best of us cannot curtail. In the end, when financial incentives guide our elderly toward a path that emphasizes palliative medical care to enhance dignity and function, rather than the precipice of high-cost medical aggression, I know that people will be happier and healthier. Clinical studies, and the whole of my experience, demonstrate that the elderly do not want to be tossed into the caldron of medical excess when intervention is hopeless. Most of my patients seek comfort in their later years. And comfort comes cheap. It is hard get rid of the medical falsehoods that are so pervasive in society. But if Medicare changed course and nudged people in a different direction, our medical landscape would be much more beautiful and affordable.

If we intelligently curb care by allowing patients to make reasonable choices, we are not only going to save Medicare, we will also be saving lives. A thorough medical system need not bankrupt the insurance that finances it. In fact, the most thorough system that we can build for our elderly would be inexpensive, humane, and lifesaving. With just a sprinkle of political will, and a whiff of common sense, the answer sits on our stoops. It is time to open up the door and take a look.

NOTES

Foreword

1. M. J. Hall, S. Levant, and C. J. DeFrances, *Trends in Inpatient Hospital Deaths: National Hospital Discharge Survey, 2000–2010,* National Center for Health Statistics data brief, no. 118 (Hyattsville, MD: National Center for Health Statistics, 2013).

2. D. C. Goodman, E. S. Fisher, J. E. Wennberg, J. S. Skinner, S. Chasan-Taber, K. K. Bronner, *Tracking Improvement in the Care of Chronically Ill Patients: A Dartmouth Atlas Brief on Medicare Beneficiaries Near the End of Life* (Lebanon, NH: Dartmouth Institute for Health Policy and Clinical Practice, 2013).

3. S. B. Hardin and Y. A. Yusufaly, "Difficult End-of-Life Treatment Decisions: Do Other Factors Trump Advance Directives?," *Arch Intern Med* 164, no. 14 (2004): 1531–33.

4. G. Easterbrook, "The Revolution in Medicine," *Newsweek,* January 26, 1987, 40–44, 49–74.

5. J. E. Wennberg, E. S. Fisher, D. C. Goodman, and J. S. Skinner, *Tracking the Care of Patients with Severe Chronic Illness,* Dartmouth Atlas of Health Care 2008 (Lebanon, NH: Dartmouth Institute for Health Policy and Clinical Practice, 2008).

6. J. E. Wennberg, *Tracking Medicine: A Researcher's Quest to Understand Health Care* (New York: Oxford University Press, 2010).

Introduction

1. J. S. Goodwin, "Geriatrics and the Limits of Modern Medicine," *New England Journal of Medicine* 340, no. 16 (1999): 1283–85.

2. Shannon Brownlee, *Overtreated: Why Too Much Medicine Is Making Us Sicker and Poorer* (New York: Bloomsbury Press, 2007), 199; L. M. Schwartz, "Enthusiasm for Cancer Screening in the United States," *Journal of the American Medical Association* 291, no. 1 (January 2004): 71–78.

3. Paul Starr, *The Social Transformation of American Medicine* (New York: Basic Books, 1982), 280–86.

4. "Doctors Question Medicare Stand; AMA Position Challenged at Rally for Eldercare," *New York Times*, February 7, 1965, 57; Donovan F. Ward, "Are 200,000 Doctors Wrong?" *Journal of the American Medical Association* 191, no. 8 (February 1965): 661–63; William P. Keim, "What the AMA Really Fears," *The New Republic,* February 13, 1965, 11; Starr, *Social Transformation*, 369–78.

5. "AMA House Backs Eldercare Program, Asks Study of Kerr-Mills Expansion," *Journal of the American Medical Association* 191, no. 8 (February 1965): 32–33; "Medicare Boycott Urged for Doctors," *New York Times*, August 5, 1965, 1; "A Doctor's Revolt in the US," *US News and World Report*, July 5, 1965, 26–28; Starr, *Social Transformation*, 376–78.

6. L. B. Srestha and E. J. Heisler, "The Changing Demographic Profile of the United States" (Congressional Research Service, 2011), 13–18, https://www.fas.org/sgp/crs/misc/rl32701.pdf.

7. "2015 Alzheimer's Disease Facts and Figures," Alzheimer's Association website, http://www.alz.org/facts/overview.asp.

8. "Costs of Alzheimer's to Medicare and Medicaid," Alzheimer's Association Fact Sheet, February 2015, http://act.alz.org/site/DocServer/2012_Costs_Fact_Sheet_version_2.pdf?docID=7161.

9. Ira Byock, *The Best Care Possible* (New York: Avery, 2012), 253.

10. "Spending Patterns for Prescription Drugs under Medicare Part D," *Economic and Budget Issue Brief CBO*, 1, https://www.cbo.gov/publication/42692.

11. John Abramson, *Overdosed America: The Broken Promise of American Medicine* (New York: Harpers, 2008), 244–49.

12. "Total Medicare Spending from 1974 to 2014," *Statista,* http://www.statista.com/248073/distribution-of-medicare-spending-by-service -type.

13. "Health Care Spending and the Medicare Program," *Medpac Data Book,* June 2015, http://www.medpac.gov/documents/data-book/june-2015-databook-health-care-spending-and-the-medicare-program.

14. S. Boodman, "The 1% Solution," *Washington Post*, October 8, 2013, E1.

15. R. S. Morrison, "When Too Much Is Too Little," *New England Journal of Medicine* 335, no. 23 (1996): 1755–59; E. S. Fisher, "Medical Care: Is More Always Better?" *New England Journal of Medicine* 349, no. 17 (2003): 1665–67.

16. M. Mitka, "Too Few Old Patients in Cancer Trials: Experts Say Disparity Affects Research Results and Care," *Journal of the American Medical Association* 290, no. 1 (August 2003): 27–28; Nortin Hadler, *Rethinking Aging* (Chapel Hill: University of North Carolina Press, 2011), 190.

17. Brownlee, *Overtreated*, 237.

18. These include Shannon Brownlee's *Overtreated*; H. Gilbert Welch's *Overdiagnosed: Making People Sick in the Pursuit of Health* (Boston: Beacon Press, 2011); Nortin Hadler's *The Last Well Person: How to Stay Well Despite the Health-Care System* (Montreal: McGill-Queens University Press, 2007) and *Rethinking Aging*; John Abramson's *Overdosed America: The Broken Promise of American Medicine* (New York: Harper Collins, 2011); Erik Rifkin and Edward Bouwer's *The Illusion of Certainty: Health Benefits and Risks* (New York: Springer Science and Media, 2007); Robert Duggan's *Breaking the Iron Triangle: Reducing Health-Care Costs in Corporate America* (Columbia, MD: Wisdom Well Press, 2012); and Byock's *Best Care Possible*, among other books that I cite extensively.

19. Abramson, *Overdosed America*, 183.

20. J. M. Teno, "Medical Care Inconsistent with Patients' Treatment Goals," *Journal of the American Geriatric Society* 50 (2002): 496–500; P. A. Singer, "Quality End-of-Life Care: Patients' Perspectives," *Journal of the American Medical Association* 281, no. 2 (January 1999): 163–68; A. E. Barnato et al., "Are Regional Variations in End-of-Life Care Intensity Explained by Patient Preferences?" *Med Care* 45 (2007): 386–93; P. Pronovost, "Economics of End-of-Life Care in the Intensive Care Unit," *Critical Care Medicine* 29, no. 2 (2001): 46–51.

21. K. T. Unroe, "Resource Use in the Last Six Months of Life among Medicare Beneficiaries with Heart Failure: 2000–7," *Archives of Internal Medicine* 171, no. 3 (2011): 196–203; Duggan, *Breaking the Iron Triangle*, 80; D. R. Hoover, "Medical Expenditures during the Last Year of Life," *Health Services Research* 37, no. 6 (2002): 1625–42; Baohui Zhang, "Health Care Costs in the Last Week of Life: Association with End-of-Life Conversations," *Archives of Internal Medicine* 169, no. 5 (2009): 480–85; J. D. Lubitz, "Trends in Medicare Payments in the Last Year of Life," *New England Journal of Medicine* 328, no. 15 (1993): 1092–96.

22. Byock, *Best Care Possible*, 3.

1. Defining Quality

1. John Abramson, *Overdosed America: The Broken Promise of American Medicine* (New York: Harpers, 2008), 247.

2. SHEP Cooperative Research Group, "Prevention of Stroke by Antihypertensive Drug Treatment in Older Persons with Isolated Systolic Hypertension," *Journal of the American Medical Association* 265, no. 24 (June 1991): 3255–64.

3. Nortin Hadler, *Rethinking Aging* (Chapel Hill: University of North Carolina Press, 2011), 13.

4. Nortin Hadler, *The Last Well Person: How to Stay Well Despite the Health-Care System* (Montreal: McGill-Queens University Press, 2007), 146.

5. Abramson, *Overdosed America*, 103.

6. B. Als-Neilson, "Association of Funding and Conclusions in Randomized Drug Trials," *Journal of the American Medical Association* 290, no. 7 (August 2003): 921–28; N. K. Chowdry, "Relationships between Authors of Clinical Practice Guidelines and the Pharmaceutical Industry," *Journal of the American Medical Association* 287, no. 5 (February 2002): 612–17; Shannon Brownlee, *Overtreated: Why Too Much Medicine Is Making Us Sicker and Poorer* (New York: Bloomsbury Press, 2007), 222–28; T. Boderheim, "Uneasy Alliance: Clinical Investigators and the Pharmaceutical Industry," *New England Journal of Medicine* 32 (2002): 1539–44; Abramson, *Overdosed America*, 115.

7. Paraphrased from the 2015 Physician Quality Reporting System Measures List, https://www.cms.gov/medicare/quality-initiatives-patient-assessment-instruments/pqrs/measurescodes.html.

8. S. H. Hohnloser, "Incidence of Stroke in Paroxysmal vs. Sustained Afib in Patients Taking Oral Anticoagulation or Combined Antiplatelet Therapy," *Journal of the American College of Cardiology* 50 (2007): 2156–61.

9. J. Mant, "Coumadin vs. Aspirin for Afib in the Elderly," *Lancet* 370 (2007): 497–51.

10. M. Ebell, "Chosing between Warfarin and Aspirin Therapy for Patients with Atrial Fibrillation," *American Family Physician* 71 no. 12 (June 2005): 2348–50.

11. S. D. Fihn, "The Risk for and Severity of Bleeding Complications in Elderly Patients Treated with Warfarin," *Annals of Internal Medicine* 124, no. 11 (1996): 970–79; T. Gomes, "Rates of Hemorrhage during Warfarin Therapy for Atrial Fibrillation," *Canadian Medical Association Journal* 185 (2013): E121–27.

12. The Stroke Prevention in Atrial Fibrillation Investigators, "Bleeding during Anti-thrombotic Therapy in Patients with Atrial Fibrillation," *Arch Intern Med* 156, no. 4 (February 26, 1996): 409–16.

13. B. F. Gage, "Risk of Osteoporotic Fracture in Elderly Patients Taking Warfarin," *Archives of Internal Medicine* 166, no. 2 (2006): 241.

14. Paraphrased from the 2015 Physician Quality Reporting System Measures List, https://www.cms.gov/medicare/quality-initiatives-patient-assessment-instruments/pqrs/measurescodes.html.

15. B. J. Powers, "Measuring Blood Pressure for Decision Making and Quarterly Reporting: Where and How Many Measures," *Annals of Internal Medicine* 154 (2011): 781–85; C. Bowron, "Better Technology Shows That Too Many People Are Treated for High Blood Pressure," *Washington Post*, June 4, 2013, E1.

16. B. Ovbiagele et al., "Level of Systolic Blood Pressure within the Normal Range and Risk of Recurrent Stroke," *Journal of the American Medical Association* 306, no. 19 (November 2011): 2137–44.

17. R. M. Cooper-DeHoff et al., "Tight Blood Pressure Control and Cardiovascular Outcomes among Hypertensive Patients with Diabetes and CAD," *Journal of the American Medical Association* 304, no. 1 (July 2010): 61–68; M. R. Law, "Use of Blood Pressure Lowering Drugs in the Prevention of Cardiovascular Disease," *BMJ* 338 (2009): 1665; F. N. Messerli, "Dogma Disputed: Can Aggressively Lowering Blood Pressure in Hypertensive Patients with CAD Be Dangerous?" *Annals of Internal Medicine* 144 (2006): 884–93.

18. C. Kovesdy, "Blood Pressure and Mortality in US Veterans with Chronic Kidney Disease," *Annals of Internal Medicine* 159, no. 4 (2013): 233–42.

19. D. Brauser, "SPRINT's Impact on BP Management: 'Groundbreaking' but Many Questions Remain," November 18, 2015, Medscape Conference News, http://www.medscape.com/viewarticle/854681?nlid=91815_2825&src=wnl_edit_medn_imed&uac=209828BG&spon=18&impID=896069&faf=1#vp_2.

20. Hadler, *Rethinking Aging*, 45, 48; F. Boutitie, "J-shaped Relationship between Blood Pressure and Mortality in Hypertensive Patients," *Annals of Internal Medicine* 136, no. 6 (2002): 438–48; M. D. Bangalor, "What Is the Optimal Blood Pressure in Patients after Acute Coronary Syndromes?" *Circulation* 122 (2010): 142–45.

21. K. Louden, "Aggressive Antihypertensive Drug Use Can Harm Elderly," Medscape, May 26, 2015, http://www.medscape.com/viewarticle/845396.

22. M. Myers, "Overtreatment of Hypertension in the Community?" *American Journal of Hypertension* 9, no. 5 (1996): 419–25; B. Lernfelt, "Overtreatment of Hypertension in the Elderly?" *Journal of Hypertension* 8, no. 5 (1990): 483–90.

23. D. A. Butt et al., "The Risk of Hip Fracture after Initiating Antihypertensive Drugs in the Elderly," *Archives of Internal Medicine* 172, no. 22 (2012): 1739–44.

24. Paraphrased from the 2015 Physician Quality Reporting System Measures List, https://www.cms.gov/medicare/quality-initiatives-patient-assessment-instruments/pqrs/measurescodes.html.

25. ADVANCE Collaborative Group, "Intense Blood Glucose Control and Vascular Outcomes in Patients with Type 2 Diabetes," *New England Journal of Medicine* 358 (2008): 2560–71; T. N. Kelly, "Systemic Review: Glucose Control and Cardiovascular Disease in Type 2 Diabetes," *Annals of Internal Medicine* 151 (2009): 394–407; W. Duckworth, "Glucose Control and Vascular Complications in Veterans with Type 2 Diabetes," *New England Journal of Medicine* 360 (2009): 129–39; M. Mitka, "Aggressive Glycemic Control Might Not Be the Best Choice for All Diabetic Patients," *Journal of the American Medical Association* 303, no. 10 (March 2010) : 1137–46; The Action to Control Cardiovascular Risk in Diabetes Study Group, "Effects of Intense Glucose Lowering in Type 2 Diabetes," *New England Journal of Medicine* 358 (2008): 2545–50.

26. R. A. Whitmer et al., "Hypoglycemic Episodes and Risk of Dementia in Patients with Type 2 Diabetes," *Journal of the American Medical Association* 301, no. 15 (April 2009): 1565–72;

C. L. Meinert, "A Study of the Effects of Hypoglycemic Agents on Vascular Complications in Patients with Adult Onset Diabetes," *Diabetes* 19 (1970): 789–830.

27. C. K. Yau, "Glycolylated Hemoglobin and Functional Decline in Community Dwelling Nursing Home Eligible Elderly Adults with Diabetes," *Journal of the American Geriatrics Society* 60 (2012): 1215–21.

28. W. Aronow, "Oral Sulfonylurea and Cardiovascular Mortality," *Geriatrics* 59, no. 9 (2004): 45; S. Simpson, "Dose-Response Relationship between Sulfonylurea Drugs and Mortality in Type 2 Diabetes: A Population Based Cohort Study," *CMAJ* 174, no. 2 (2006): 169–74; Hadler, *Rethinking Aging*, 34–37; L. L. Lipscombe et al., "Thiazolidinediones and Cardiovascular Outcomes in Older Patients with Diabetes," *Journal of the American Medical Association* 298, no. 22 (December 2007): 2634–43.

29. Paraphrased from the 2015 Physician Quality Reporting System Measures List, https://www.cms.gov/medicare/quality-initiatives-patient-assessment-instruments/pqrs/measurescodes.html.

30. J. Kastelen, "Simvastatin with or without Ezetimine in Familial Hypercholesterolemia," *New England Journal of Medicine* 358 (2008): 1431–43.

31. J. Dach, "Cholesterol Lowering Drugs for the Elderly, a Very Bad Idea," 2008, http://www.drdach.com/cholesterol_statin_elderly.html; E. Rifkin and E. Bouwer, *The Illusion of Certainty: Health Benefits and Risks* (New York: Springer Science and Media, 2007), 89.

32. Abramson, *Overdosed America*, 14–16, 145; Hadler, *Last Well Person*, 36; Hadler, *Rethinking Aging*, 28; Z. Reiner, "Statins in the Primary Prevention of Cardiovascular Disease," *National Review of Cardiology* 10, no. 8 (2013): 453–64; K. Louden, "Statins Questionable for Elderly Men without Heart Disease," Medscape, May 28, 2015, http://www.medscape.com/viewarticle/845517.

33. Michael O'Riordan, "New Cholesterol Guidelines Abandon LDL Targets," Medscape, November 14, 2013, http://www.medscape.com/viewarticle/814152.

34. Paraphrased from the 2015 Physician Quality Reporting System Measures List, https://www.cms.gov/medicare/quality-initiatives-patient-assessment-instruments/pqrs/measurescodes.html.

35. Hadler, *Rethinking Aging*, 121; Hadler, *Last Well Person*, 162; Abramson, *Overdosed America*, 213; H. Gilbert Welch, *Overdiagnosed: Making People Sick in the Pursuit of Health* (Boston: Beacon Press, 2011), 27.

36. G. A. Wells et al., "Alendronate for the Primary and Secondary Prevention of Osteoporotic Fractures in Postmenopausal Women," Cochrane Database of Systematic Review, 2008.

37. J. P. Schneider, "Bisphosphonates and Low-Impact Femoral Fractures: Current Evidence on Alendronate Fracture Risk," *Geriatrics* 64, no. 1 (January 2009): 18–23.

38. Brownlee, *Overtreated*, 181.

39. Paraphrased from the 2015 Physician Quality Reporting System Measures List, https://www.cms.gov/medicare/quality-initiatives-patient-assessment-instruments/pqrs/measurescodes.html.

40. Abramson, *Overdosed America*, 104.

41. J. Birks, "Cholinesterase Inhibitors for Alzheimer's Disease," *Cochrane Database Syst Rev.* 2006; H. Kavirajan, "Efficacy and Adverse Effects of Cholinesterase Inhibitors and Memantine in Vascular Dementia: A Meta-Analysis of Randomised Controlled Trials," *Lancet Neurology*, no. 9 (September 6, 2007): 782–92; B. Winblad, "A 1-Year, Randomized, Placebo-Controlled Study of Donepezil in Patients with Mild to Moderate AD," *Neurology* 57 (2001): 489–95.

42. R. Howard, "Donepezil and Memantine for Moderate Severe Alzheimer's Disease," *New England Journal of Medicine* 366 (2012): 893–903.

43. K. Lanctôt et al., "Efficacy and Safety of Cholinesterase Inhibitors in Alzheimer's Disease: A Meta-analysis," *CMAJ* 169, no. 6 (September 16, 2003): 557–64.

44. P. Raina, "Effectiveness of Cholinesterase Inhibitors and Memantine for Treating Dementia: Evidence Review for a Clinical Practice Guideline," *Annals of Internal Medicine* 148, no. 5 (March 4, 2008): 379–97.

45. L. Schneider, "Lack of Evidence for the Efficacy of Memantine in Mild Alzheimer Disease," *Arch Neurol* 68, no. 8 (2011): 991–98; S. A. Areosa, "Memantine for Dementia," *Cochrane Database Syst Rev.* 3 (2005); L. Searing, "A Daily Dose of Vitamin E May Slow Early Alzheimer's Disease," *Washington Post*, January 4, 2014, E3. This study compared vitamin E to Namenda, and found that Namenda had no impact on function while vitamin E did.

46. R. Howard, "Donepezil and Memantine for Moderate Severe Alzheimer's Disease," *New England Journal of Medicine* 366 (2012): 893–903.

47. L. E. Middleton, "Activity Energy Expenditure and Incident of Cognitive Impairment in Older Adults," *Archives of Internal Medicine* 171, no. 14 (2011): 1251–57; E. B. Russian, "Exercise Is Associated with Reduced Risk for Incident Dementia among Persons 64 Years Old and Older," *Annals of Internal Medicine* 144 (2006): 73–81; D. Laurin, "Physical Activity and Risk of Cognitive Impairment and Dementia in Elderly Persons," *Archives of Neurology* 58 (2001): 498–504; Hadler, *Rethinking Aging*, 168.

48. Alliance for Human Research Protection, "Petition to FDA: Withdraw Aricept 23 mg Immediately," http://www.ahrp.org/cms/content/view/813/56. Other studies cited show the high side effect profile and dropout rate.

49. S. Gill, "Syncope and Its Consequences in Patients with Dementia Receiving Cholinesterase Inhibitors," *Archives of Internal Medicine* 169, no. 86 (2009): 7–73.

50. Brownlee, *Overtreated,* 186; J. Donohue, "A Decade of Direct-to-Consumer Advertising of Prescription Drugs," *New England Journal of Medicine* 357 (2007): 673–81.

51. J. P. Orlowski, "The Effects of Pharmaceutical Firms on Physician Prescribing Patterns," *Chest* 102 (1992): 270–77; J. Dana and G. Lowenstein, "A Social Science Perspective on Gifts to Physicians from Industry," *Journal of the American Medical Association* 290, no. 2 (July 2003): 252–55; A. Wazana "Physicians and the Pharmaceutical Industry: Is a Gift Ever Just a Gift?," *Journal of the American Medical Association* 283, no. 3 (January 2000): 373–80.

52. Abramson, *Overdosed America*, 105.

53. F. Adair, "Do Drug Samples Influence Resident Prescribing Behavior?" *American Journal of Medicine* 118 (2005): 881–84.

54. Abramson, *Overdosed America*, 101.

55. Brownlee, *Overtreated,* 219.

56. Yu-xio Yang, "Long Term Proton Pump Inhibitor Therapy and Risk of Hip Fracture," *Journal of the American Medical Association* 296, no. 24 (December 2006): 2947–53; S. J. Diem, "Use of Antidepressants and Rate of Hip Bone Loss in Older Women," *Archives of Internal Medicine* 167, no. 12 (2007): 1240–45; Hadler, *Rethinking Aging*, 165.

57. HOPE-TOO Trial Investigators, "Long Term Vitamin E Supplements in Patients with Vascular Disease or Diabetes," *Journal of the American Medical Association* 293, no. 11 (March 2005): 1338–47; C. M. Albert, "Effect of Folic Acid and B Vitamins on Risk of Cardiovascular Events and Total Mortality among Females at High Risk for Cardiovascular Disease," *Journal of the American Medical Association* 299, no. 17 (May 2008): 2027–36; S. K. Myung, "Efficacy of Vitamin and Antioxidant Supplements in Prevention of Cardiovascular Disease," *BMJ* 346 (2013): F10; E. A. Klein, "Vitamin E and the Risk of Prostate Cancer: The Selenium and Vitamin E Cancer Prevention Trial," *Journal of the American Medical Association* 306, no. 14 (October 2011): 1549–55.

58. L. Searing, "A Daily Dose of Vitamin E May Slow Early Alzheimer's Disease," *Washington Post*, January 4, 2014, E3.

59. E. Ernst, "The Risk-Benefit Profile of Commonly Used Herbal Therapies," *Annals of Internal Medicine* 136, no. 1 (2002): 42–53.

60. M. J. Bolland, "Vascular Events in Healthy Older Women Receiving Calcium Supplementation," *BMJ* 336 (2008), http://www.bmj.com/content/336/7638/262; Hadler, *Last Well Person*, 154; E. Seeman, "Evidence That Calcium Supplements Reduce Fracture Risk Is Lacking," *Clin J Am Soc Nephrol* 5 (January 2010): S53–11; M. J. Bolland, "Calcium Supplements and Fracture Prevention," *New England Journal of Medicine* 370 (2014): 386–88; M. J. Bolland et al., "Calcium Supplements with or without Vitamin D and Risk of Cardiovascular Events: Reanalysis of the Women's Health Initiative," *BMJ* 342 (2011), http://www.bmj.com/content/342/bmj.d2040; M. J. Bolland et al., "Calcium Intake and Risk of Fracture: Systemic Review," *BMJ* 315 (2015): 4580; Vicky Tai et al., "Calcium Intake and Bone Mineral Denisty: Systemic Review and Meta-analysis," *BMJ* 315 (2015): 4183.

61. S. Kwak, "Efficacy of Omega-3 Fatty Acid Supplements in the Secondary Prevention of Cardiovascular Disease," *Archives of Internal Medicine* 175, no. 9 (2012): 686–94; Risk and Prevention Study Collaborative Group, "N-3 Fatty Acids in Patients with Multiple Cardiovascular Risk Factors," *New England Journal of Medicine* 368 (2013): 1800–1808; T. M. Brasky, "Plasma Phospholipid Fatty Acids and Prostate Cancer Risk in the SELECT Trial," *Journal of the National Cancer Institute* 105 no. 15 (2013): 1132–41. Multiple trials of omega-3 acids have been conducted with varying results, some of which have different doses and examine different populations. None show dramatic improvement, but some do show a cardiac benefit in certain circumstances.

62. S. R. Seshasai, "Effect of Aspirin on Vascular and Nonvascular Outcomes: Meta-analysis of Randomized Controlled Trials," *Archives of Internal Medicine* 172, no. 3 (2012): 206–16.

63. Eliseo Guallar, "Enough Is Enough: Stop Wasting Money on Vitamin and Mineral Supplements," *Annals of Internal Medicine* 159, no. 12 (December 17, 2013): 850–1. See accompanying studies in the same issue that look in depth at multivitamin supplementation; J. Mursu, "Dietary Supplements and Mortality Rate in Older Women: The Iowa Women's Health Study," *Archives of Internal Medicine* 171, no. 18 (2011): 1625–33; D. M. Quato et al., "Use of Prescription and OTC Medicines and Dietary Supplements among Older Adults in the United States," *Journal of the American Medical Association* 300, no. 24 (December 2008): 2867–78; G. Bjelakovic et al., "Mortality in Randomized Trials of Antioxidant Supplements for Primary and Secondary Prevention," *Journal of the American Medical Association* 297, no. 8 (February 2007): 842–57; A. Cha, "Study Questions Antioxidant Use in Cancer Patients," *Washington Post*, January 30, 2014, A2; G. Bjelakovic, "Antioxidant Supplements to Prevent Mortality," *Journal of the American Medical Association* 310, no. 11 (September 2013): 1178–79; Heart Protection Study Collaboration Group. "MRC/BHF Heart Protection Study of Antioxidant Vitamin Supplementation in 20 536 High-Risk Individuals: A Randomised Placebo-Controlled Trial," *Lancet* 360 (2002): 23–33.

64. T. J. Kaptchuck, "Placebo without Deception," *Plosone*, 2010, http://www.plosone.org/article/info%3Adoi%2F10.1371%2Fjournal.pone.0015591.

65. Marta Peciña et al., "Association between Placebo-Activated Neural Systems and Antidepressant Responses," *JAMA Psychiatry,* September 30, 2015, doi:10.1001/jamapsychiatry.2015.1335.

66. B. Barrett, "Placebo Effects and the Common Cold: A Randomized Controlled Trial," *Annals of Family Medicine* 9 (2011): 312–27.

67. Abramson, *Overdiagnosed America,* 127, 140.

68. E. Guallar, "Controversy over Clinical Guidelines: Listen to the Evidence, Not the Noise," *Annals of Internal Medicine* 160, no. 5 (March 4, 2014): 361–62.

69. See, for example, a list of guidelines from Kaiser's Ohio group, http://providers.kaiserpermanente.org/oh/clinicalguidelines.html.

70. Available in the Northern Maryland Collaborative Care handbook.

71. J. H. Gurwitz, "Incidence and Preventability of Adverse Drug Events among Older Persons," *Journal of the American Medical Association* 289, no. 9 (March 2003): 1107–16; R. Voelker,

"Common Drugs Can Harm Elderly Patients," *Journal of the American Medical Association* 302, no. 6 (August 2009): 614–15; P. Routledge, "Adverse Drug Reactions in Elderly Patients," *British Journal of Clinical Pharmacology* 57, no. 2 (2004): 121–26; J. F. Kurfees, "Drug Interactions in the Elderly," *Journal of Family Practice* 25, no. 5 (1987): 471–85.

72. Brownlee, *Overtreatment*, 274.

2. Defining Thorough

1. B. Starfield, "Is US Health Really the Best in the World?" *Journal of the American Medical Association* 284, no. 4 (July 2000): 483–85; R. A. Deyo, "Cascade Effects of Medical Technology," *Annual Review of Public Health* 23 (2002): 23–44.

2. Shannon Brownlee, *Overtreated* (New York: Bloomsbury Press, 2007), 158.

3. Ibid., 144.

4. H. Gilbert Welch, *Overdiagnosed: Making People Sick in the Pursuit of Health* (Boston: Beacon Press, 2011), 35.

5. Brownlee, *Overtreated*, 105.

6. See especially Welch, *Overdiagnosed*; E. Rifkin and E. Bouwer, *The Illusion of Certainty: Health Benefits and Risks* (New York: Springer Science and Media, 2007).

7. B. Davies, "Rethinking the Value of the Annual Exam," *ACP Internist*, January 2010. Many other experts are questioning the value of a complete exam, which Erik Rifkin and I discuss in *Interpreting Health Benefits and Risks: A Practical Guide to Facilitate Doctor-Patient Communication* (New York: Springer, 2014).

8. Nortin Hadler, *Rethinking Aging* (Chapel Hill: University of North Carolina Press, 2011), 67.

9. Welch, *Overdiagnosed*, 49.

10. G. L. Andriole, "Mortality Results from a Randomized Prostate Cancer Screening Trial," *New England Journal of Medicine* 360 (2009): 1310–19; H. G. Welch, "Prostate Cancer Diagnosis and Treatment after the Introduction of PSA Screening, 1986–2005," *Journal of National Cancer Institute* 101, no. 19 (2009): 1325–29; Brownlee, *Overtreated*, 200; K. Lin, "Benefits and Harms of PSA Screening for Prostate Cancer: An Evidence Update for the US Preventive Task Force," *Annals of Internal Medicine* 149 (2008): 192–99.

11. Lin, "Benefits and Harms of PSA Screening."

12. E. A. M. Heijnsdijk, "Quality of Life Effect of Prostate-Specific Antigen Screening," *New England Journal of Medicine* 367 (2012): 595–605; F. Fang, "Immediate Risk for Cardiovascular Events and Suicide Following a Prostate Cancer Diagnosis," *Journal of National Cancer Institute* 102, no. 5 (2010): 307–14; D. P. Smith, "Quality of Life Three Years after Diagnosis of Localized Prostate Cancer," *BMJ* 339 (2009), http://www.ncbi.nlm.nih.gov/pubmed/19945997.

13. Nortin Hadler, *The Last Well Person: How to Stay Well Despite the Health-Care System* (Montreal: McGill-Queens University Press, 2007), 99.

14. Welch, *Overdiagnosed*; Hadler, *Last Well Person*; and John Abramson, *Overdosed America: The Broken Promise of American Medicine* (New York: Harpers, 2008), all talk about the inability of cancer treatment to extend life for elderly patients.

15. "Recommendations for Primary Care Practice," US Preventive Services Task Force, http://www.uspreventiveservicestaskforce.org/Page/Name/recommendations.

16. A. Bleyer, "Effect of Three Decades of Screening Mammograms on Breast Cancer Incidence," *New England Journal of Medicine* 367 (2012): 1998–2005.

17. H. G. Welch, "Over Diagnosis of Mammogram Screening: The Question of Not Whether but How Often It Occurs," *BMJ* 339 (2009): 182–83; H. G. Welch, "Screening Mammography: A Long Run for a Short Ride," *New England Journal of Medicine* 363 (2010): 1276–80; K. A. Phillips,

"Putting the Risk of Breast Cancer into Perspective," *New England Journal of Medicine* 340, no. 2 (1999): 141–44; D. H. Zahl, "The Natural History of Invasive Breast Cancer Detected by Screening Mammography," *Archives of Internal Medicine* 168, no. 21 (2008): 2311–15.

18. G. Kolata, "Vast Study Casts Doubt on Value of Mammogram," *New York Times*, February 11, 2014, http://www.nytimes.com/2014/02/12/health/study-adds-new-doubts-about-value-of-mammograms.html?_r=0.

19. H. Welch, "Breast Cancer Screenings: What We Still Don't Know," *New York Times*, December 30, 2013.

20. B. Monsees, "Weighing the Value of Mammogram," *New York Times*, January 2, 2014.

21. L. Walter, "Cancer Screening in Elderly Patients," *Journal of the American Medical Association* 285, no. 21 (June 2001): 2750–56.

22. R. Smith-Bindman, "Is Screening Mammography Effective in Elderly Women?" *American Journal of Medicine* 108, no. 2 (February 2000): 112–19.

23. C. Lerman, "Psychological and Behavior Implications of Abnormal Mammograms," *Annals of Internal Medicine* 114, no. 8 (1991): 657–61; N. T. Brewer, "The Long Term Effects of False Positive Mammograms," *Annals of Internal Medicine* 146, no. 7 (2007): 502–10.

24. Tara Parker-Pope, "New Cautions About Longer-term Use of Bone Drugs," *The New York Times,* May 9, 2012, http://well.blogs.nytimes.com/2012/05/09/new-cautions-about-long-term-use-of-bone-drugs/?_r=0.; "What's the Story with Fosamax?" Harvard Women's Health Watch, November 1, 2008, http://www.health.harvard.edu/newsletters/Harvard_Womens_Health_Watch/2008/November/Whats_the_story_with_Fosamax. See also references from chapter 1 about Fosamax.

25. Brownlee, *Overtreated*, 213.

26. M. L. Gourlay, "Bone Density Testing Intervals and Transition to Osteoporosis in Older Women," *New England Journal of Medicine* 366 (2012): 225–32.

27. M. B. Herndon, "Implications of Expanded Disease Definitions: The Case of Osteoporosis," *Health Affairs* 26 (2007): 1702–11.

28. Hadler, *Last Well Person*, 72.

29. P. Span, "Too Many Colonoscopies in the Elderly," *New York Times*, March 12, 2013; J. Wilson, "Colon Cancer Screening in the Elderly: When Do We Stop?" *Transactions of the American Clinical and Climatological Association* 121 (2010): 94–103.

30. V. Pastorino, "Early Lung Cancer Detection with Spiral CT and Positron Emission Tomography in Heavy Smokers: 2 Year Results," *Lancet* 362 (2003): 593–97.

31. NLST Research Team, "Reduced Lung-Cancer Mortality with Low-Dose CT Screening," *New England Journal of Medicine* 365 (2011): 395–409.

32. H. De Koning, "Benefits and Harms of Computed Tomography Lung Cancer Screening Strategies: A Comparative Modeling Study for the US Preventive Services Task Force," *Annals of Internal Medicine* 160, no. 5 (March 4, 2014): 311–20.

33. E. F. Patz, "Overdiagnosis in Low-Dose Computed Tomography Screening for Lung Cancer," *JAMA Internal Medicine* 174, no. 2 (February 1, 2014): 269–74.

34. A. Fein, "Clinical Practice: The Solitary Pulmonary Nodule," *New England Journal of Medicine* 348 (2003): 2535–47; H. MacMahon, "Guidelines for Management of Small Pulmonary Nodules Detected on CT Scans," *Radiology* 237 (2005): 395–406; Welch, *Overdiagnosed*, 67; H. G. Welch, "Overdiagnosis in Cancer," *Journal of the National Cancer Institute* 102, no. 9 (May 5, 2010): 605–13.

35. A. Berrington de Gonzalez, "Low Dose Lung CT Screening before Age 55: Estimates of the Mortality Reduction Required to Outweigh the Radiation-Induced Cancer Risk," *J Med Screening* 15, no. 3 (2008): 153–58.

36. P. Hahn, editorial, *Baltimore Sun*, March 29, 2013, 17.

37. Welch, *Overdiagnosed,* 144.

38. Hadler, *Rethinking Aging*, 50.

39. Welch, *Overdiagnosed*, 114.

40. Brownlee, *Overtreated*, 150, 158, 166.

41. Welch, *Overdiagnosed*, 36.

42. O. Bruyere, "Radiologic Features Poorly Predict Clinical Outcome in Knee Osteoarthritis," *Scandinavian Journal of Rheumatology* 31, no. 1 (2002): 13–16; M. Englund, "Incidental Meniscal Findings on Knee MRI in Middle Age and Elderly Persons," *New England Journal of Medicine* 359 (2008): 1108–15.

43. R. Redberg, "We Are Giving Ourselves Cancer," *New York Times*, January 31, 2014, A27.

44. Welch, *Overdiagnosed*, 47.

45. Brownlee, *Overtreated*, 149.

46. J. Jarvik, "Diagnostic Evaluation of Lower Back Pain with Emphasis on Imaging," *Annals of Internal Medicine* 37, no. 7 (2002): 586–97; B. Roudsari, "Lumbar Spine MRI for Low Back Pain: Indications and Yield," *American Journal of Roentgenology* 195, no. 3 (2010): 550–59; A. El Barzouhi, "Magnetic Resonance Imaging in Follow-up Assessment of Sciatica," *New England Journal of Medicine* 368 (2013): 999–1007.

47. R. Chou, "Diagnostic Imaging for Low Back Pain: Advice for High-Value Health Care from the American College of Physicians," *Annals of Internal Medicine* 154, no. 3 (February 1, 2011): 181–89.

48. L. H. Pengel, "Acute Low Back Pain: Systematic Review of Its Prognosis," *BMJ* 327 (2003): 327.

49. R. Chou, "Imaging Strategies for Low-Back Pain: Systematic Review and Meta-analysis," *Lancet* 373 (2009): 463–72; B. S. Webster, "Relationship of Early Magnetic Resonance Imaging for Work-Related Acute Low Back Pain with Disability and Medical Utilization Outcomes," *Journal of Occupational and Environmental Medicine* 52 (2010): 900–907.

50. M. C. Jensen, "MRI of the Lumbar Spine in People without Back Pain," *New England Journal of Medicine* 331 (1994): 69–78; T. Videman, "Associations between Back Pain History and Lumbar MRI Findings," *Spine* 28, no. 6 (2003): 582–88.

51. H. J. Choi, "Epidural Steroid Injection Therapy for Lower Back Pain," *International Journal of Technology Assessment in Health Care* 29, no. 3 (2013): 244–53; R. Chou, "Surgery for Lower Back Pain: A Review of the Evidence for an American Pain Society Clinical Practice Guideline," *Spine* 34, no. 10 (2009): 1094–1109.

52. K. Radcliff, "Epidural Steroid Injections Are Associated with Less Improvement in Patients with Lumbar Spinal Stenosis: A Subgroup Analysis of the Spine Patient Outcomes Research Trial," *Spine* 38, no. 4 (2013): 279–91.

53. J. Brody, "The Treadmill's Place in Evaluating Hearts," *New York Times*, July 29, 2008.

54. A. Arbab-Saden, "Stress Testing and Non-invasive Coronary Angiography in Patients with Suspected Coronary Artery Disease," *Heart International* 7, no. 1 (February 2012): e2.

55. S. Capewell, "Will Screening Individuals High Risk of Cardiovascular Events Deliver Large Benefits?" *BMJ* 337 (2005): 783, which is a medical repudiation of an article stating the opposite.

56. David A. Fein, MD, "Was Your Stress Test the Wrong Test?," The Princeton Longevity Center Medical News, http://www.theplc.net/Cardiac_Stress_Tests.html.

57. M. Budoff and K. Gul, "Expert Review on Coronary Calcium," *Vascular Health and Risk Management* 4, no. 2 (April 2008): 315–24.

58. J. Skinner, "Is Technological Change in Medicine Always Worth It? The Case of Myocardial Infarction," *Health Affairs* 25, no. 2 (2006): w34–47.

59. J. Tu, "Use of Cardiac Procedures and Outcomes in Elderly Patients with Myocardial Infarction in the United States and Canada," *New England Journal of Medicine* 336 (1997): 1500–1505.

60. Abramson, *Overdosed America*, 172.

61. Brownlee, *Overtreated*, 99.

62. W. E. Boden, "Optimal Medical Therapy with or without PCI for Stable CAD," *New England Journal of Medicine* 356 (2007): 1503–16, shows that adding revascularization to medicines and lifestyle changes does not improve outcomes. M. Pfisterer, "Outcomes of Elderly Patients with Chronic Symptomatic Coronary Artery Disease with an Invasive vs. Optimized Medical Treatment Strategy," *Journal of the American Medical Association* 289, no. 9 (March 2003): 1117–23; R. A. Henderson, "Seven-Year Outcome in the RITA-2 Trial: Coronary Angioplasty vs. Medical Therapy," *Journal of the American College of Cardiology* 42 (2003): 1161–70.

63. Hadler, *Last Well Person*, 27–29; Brownlee, *Overtreated*, 101–2; Hadler, *Rethinking Aging*, 54–55; Abramson, *Overdosed America,* 172.

64. M. F. Newman, "Longitudinal Assessment of Neurocognitive Function after Coronary Artery Bypass Surgery," *New England Journal of Medicine* 344 (2002): 395–402.

65. B. Thorsteinsdottir, "Dialysis in the Frail Elderly: A Current Ethical Problem, an Impending Ethical Crisis," *Journal of General Internal Medicine* 28, no. 11 (2013): 1511–16; M. K. Tamura, "Functional Status of Elderly Adults before and after Initiation of Dialysis," *New England Journal of Medicine* 361 (2009): 1539–47, showing a substantial decline in the status of nursing home residents on dialysis; R. Arnold, "Dialysis in Frail Elders: A Role for Palliative Care," *New England Journal of Medicine* 361 (2009): 1597–98.

66. N. A. Black, "The Effectiveness of Surgery for Stress Incontinence in Women," *British Journal of Urology* 78, no. 4 (1996): 497–510.

67. *Tell Me More*, National Public Radio, August 14, 2013.

68. A. M. Clarfield, "The Decreasing Prevalence of Reversible Dementias: An Updated Meta-analysis," *Archives of Internal Medicine* 163, no. 18 (2003): 2219–29.

3. Excessive Specialization, Expectation, and Litigation

1. A. Gawande, "Overkill," *The New Yorker*, May 11, 2015.

2. B. Starfield, "The Effects of Specialist Supply on Populations' Health," *Health Affairs* (2005): 97–107.

3. J. Macinko, B. Starfield, and L. Shi, "Quantifying the Health Benefit of Primary Care Physician Supply in the United States," *International Journal of Health Services* 37, no. 1 (2007): 111–26.

4. J. E. Wennberg, "Executive Summary of Tracking the Care of Patients with Severe Chronic Illness: The Dartmouth Atlas of Health Care 2008," Hanover, NH: Dartmouth Institute for Policy and Clinical Practice, Center for Health Policy Research.

5. Shannon Brownlee, *Overtreated: Why Too Much Medicine Is Making Us Sicker and Poorer* (New York: Bloomsbury Press, 2007),. 36. See also J. E. Wennberg, "Geography and the Debate over Medicare Reform," *Health Affairs*, 2002.

6. Brownlee, *Overtreated,* 63, 67; Roni Rabin, "Hospitalized Patients Too Often Have No Single Physician in Charge of Their Care," *Washington Post*, April 29, 2013, E5.

7. E. Fernandez, "Aggressive Surgery for Nonfatal Skin Cancers Might Not Be Best for All Elderly Patients," University of California San Francisco News Center, April 29, 2013, http://www.ucsf.edu/news/2013/04/105436/surgery-nonfatal-skin-cancers-might-not-be-best-elderly-patients.

8. E. Rosenthal, "Patients' Costs Skyrocket; Specialists' Incomes Soar," *New York Times*, January 18, 2014.

9. R. Deyo, *Watch Your Back: How the Back Pain Industry Is Costing Us More and Giving Us Less* (Ithaca, NY: Cornell University Press, 2014).

10. T. Carey, "The Outcomes and Costs of Care for Acute Low Back Pain among Patients Seen by Primary Care Practitioners, Chiropractors, and Orthopedic Surgeons," *New England Journal of Medicine* 333 (1995): 913–17.

11. E. Rosenthal, "The $2.7 Trillion Medical Bill," *New York Times*, June 1, 2013.

12. Nortin Hadler, *Rethinking Aging* (Chapel Hill: University of North Carolina Press, 2011), 187; Brownlee, *Overtreatment*, 81.

13. John Abramson, *Overdosed America: The Broken Promise of American Medicine* (New York: Harpers, 2008), 50.

14. M. Jacobson, "Does Reimbursement Influence Chemotherapy Treatment for Cancer Patients?" *Health Affairs* 25, no. 2 (2006): 437–43; J. Erikson, "Oncologists Cutting Back in Face of New Medicare Payment Formula," *Oncology Times* 26, no. 4 (2004): 4–8.

15. Abramson, *Overdosed America*, 83.

16. Brownlee, *Overtreated*, 153, 265.

17. M. Compton, "Changes in US Medical Students' Specialty Interests over the Course of Medical School," *Journal of General Internal Medicine* 23, no. 7 (2008): 1095–1100.

18. T. Bodenhemer, "Primary Care: Will It Survive?" *New England Journal of Medicine* 355 (2006): 861–63.

19. G. Brandon, "How Medical Schools Consistently Cover Up Their Primary Care Failures," *Medical Economics*, May 28, 2013.

20. Brownlee, *Overtreated*, 259; S. D. Block, "Academia's Chilly Climate for Primary Care," *JAMA* 206 (1996): 677–82; D. A. Newton, "Trends in Career Choice by US Medical Schools," *JAMA* 209 (2007): 1179–82.

21. Brownlee, *Overtreated*, 259.

22. "Medscape Physician Compensation Report: 2012 Results," Medscape Multispecialty, http://www.medscape.features/slideshow/compensation/2012.

23. P. McGann, "Quality Improvement Initiatives and Tools" (lecture, AMDA conference, March 23, 2013).

24. B. Glenn, "Why Aren't Primary Care Physicians More Ticked Off about the RUC?" *Medical Economics*, April 30, 2013.

25. P. Whoriskey, "Medical Panel Uses Data That Distorts Doctors' Pay," *Washington Post*, July 21, 2013, 1.

26. "Medscape Physician Compensation Report 2015," Medscape, http://www.medscape.com/features/slideshow/compensation/2015/public/overview.

27. D. M. Studert, "Claims, Errors, and Compensatory Payments in Malpractice Litigation," *New England Journal of Medicine* 354 (2006): 2024–33; N. Kahn-Fogel, "Hanging in the Balance: Health Dogma and the Debate over Malpractice Reform," *Journal of the National Medical Association* 102, no. 3 (2010): 254–56; D. Golann, "Dropped Medical Malpractice Claims: Their Surprising Frequency, Apparent Causes and Potential Remedies," *Health Affairs* 30, no. 7 (2011): 1343–50.

28. E. Carrier, "High Physician Concern about Malpractice Risk Predicts More Aggressive Diagnostic Testing in Office-Based Practice," *Health Affairs* 32, no. 8 (2013): 1383–91; C. S. Weisman, "Practice Changes in Response to the Malpractice Litigation Climate: Results of a Physician Survey," *Medical Care* 27, no. 1 (1989): 16–24; D. Studdart, "Defensive Medicine among High-Risk Specialist Physicians in a Volatile Malpractice Environment," *JAMA* 295, no. 21 (2005): 2609–17.

29. D. Katz, "Emergency Physicians Fear of Malpractice in Evaluating Patients with Possible Acute Cardiac Ischemia," *Annals of Emergency Medicine* 46, no. 6 (2005): 525–33; G. L. Birbeck, "Do Malpractice Concerns, Payment Mechanisms, and Attitudes Influence Test Ordering Decisions?" *Neurology* 62, no. 1 (2004): 119–21.

30. A. H. Krist, "How Physicians Approach Prostate Cancer before and after Losing a Law Suit," *Annals of Family Medicine* 5 (2007): 120–27.

31. D. Klingman, "Measuring Defensive Medicine Using Clinical Scenario Surveys," *Journal of Health Politics, Policy, and Law* (1996): 185–217.

32. D. A. Hyman and C. Silver, "The Poor State of Health Care Quality in the US: Is Malpractice Liability Part of the Problem or Part of the Solution?" *Cornell Law Review* 90, no. 4 (May 2005): 896–906.

33. S. Seabury, "On Average, Physicians Spend Nearly 11% of Their 40 Year Careers with an Open, Unresolved Malpractice Claim," *Health Affairs* 32, no. 1 (2013): 111–15.

34. A. Kesselheim, "Characteristics of Physicians Who Frequently Act as Expert Witnesses in Neurologic Birth Injury Litigation," *Obstetrics and Gynecology* 108, no. 2 (2006): 273–79.

35. M. Weintraub, "Expert Witness Testimony: An Update," *Neurology Clinics* 17, no. 2 (1999): 363–69.

36. S. Paul, "States, Physician Organizations, Courts Take on Unethical Medical Experts," *American Academy of Pediatrics News* 34, no. 2 (2013): 20.

4. Hospitalization

1. "Medicare Fast Facts," National Committee to Preserve Social Security and Medicare, http://www.ncpssm.org/medicare/medicarefastfacts.

2. "The Medicare Beneficiary Population," AARP Public Policy Institute, http://assets.aarp.org/rgcenter/health/fs149_medicare.pdf.

3. Shannon Brownlee, *Overtreated: Why Too Much Medicine Is Making Us Sicker and Poorer* (New York: Bloomsbury Press, 2007), 47, 52; L. Kohn, *To Err Is Human: Building a Safer Health System* (Washington, DC: National Academy Press, 2000), 1–8.

4. W. J. Ehlenbach, "Association between Acute Care and Critical Illness Hospitalization and Cognitive Function in Older Adults," *Journal of the American Medical Association* 303, no. 8 (February 2010): 763–67; J. Witlox, "Delirium in Elderly Patients and the Risk of Postdischarge Mortality, Institutionalization, and Dementia: A Meta-analysis," *Journal of the American Medical Association* 304, no. 4 (July 2010): 443–51.

5. H. Wunsch, "Three-Year Outcomes for Medicare Beneficiaries Who Survive Intensive Care," *Journal of the American Medical Association* 303, no. 9 (March 2010): 849–60; L. Walter, "Development and Validation of a Prognostic Index for Mortality in Older Adults after Hospitalization," *Journal of the American Medical Association* 285, no. 23 (June 2001): 2987–94; Nortin Hadler, *Rethinking Aging* (Chapel Hill: University of North Carolina Press, 2011), 193.

6. D. E. Meier, "High Short-Term Mortality in Hospitalized Patients with Advanced Dementia: Lack of Benefit of Tube Feeding," *Archives of Internal Medicine* 164, no. 4 (2001): 594–99.

7. L. H. Curtis, "Early and Long-Term Outcome of Heart Failure in Elderly Persons, 2001–05," *Archives of Internal Medicine* 168, no. 22 (2008): 2481–85.

8. C. Pedone, "Elderly Patients with Cognitive Impairment Have a High Risk for Functional Decline during Hospitalization," *Journals of Gerontology Series A: Biological Sciences and Medical Sciences* 60, no. 12 (2005): 1576–80.

9. C. Morton, "Hazards of Hospitalization of the Elderly," *Annals of Internal Medicine* 118, no. 3 (1993): 219–23; K. E. Covinsky, "Loss of Independence in Activities of Daily Living in Older Adults Hospitalized with Medical Illness: Increased Vulnerability with Age," *Journal of the American Geriatrics Society* 51 (2003): 451–58; T. M. Gill, "Hospitalization, Restricted Activity, and the Development of Disability among Older Persons," *Journal of the American Medical Association* 292, no. 17 (November 2004): 2115–20.

10. C. Quach, "Risk of Infection Following a Visit to the Emergency Department: A Cohort Study," *Canadian Medical Association Journal* 184 (2012): E232–39.

11. L. Bernstein, "1 in 25 Hospital Patients Gets an Infection during Treatment, CDC Reports," *Washington Post*, March 27, 2014, A3.

12. R. Duggan, *Breaking the Iron Triangle: Reducing Health-Care Costs in Corporate America* (Columbia, MD: Wisdom Well Press, 2012), 77.

13. R. L. Kruse, "Does Hospitalization Impact Survival after Lower Respiratory Infection in Nursing Home Residents?" *Medical Care* 42 (2004): 860–70; M. Loeb, "Effect of a Clinical Pathway to Reduce Hospitalization in Nursing Home Residents with Pneumonia," *Journal of the American Medical Association* 295, no. 21 (June 2006): 2503–10; J. L. Givens, "Survival and Comfort after Treatment of Pneumonia in Advanced Dementia," *Archives of Internal Medicine* 171, no. 3 (2011): 217.

14. I. Byock, *The Best Care Possible* (New York: Avery, 2012), 107–9.

15. W. T. Longstrot, "Intravenous Tissue Plasminogen Activator and Stroke in the Elderly," *American Journal of Emergency Medicine* 28, no. 3 (2010): 359–63.

16. G. Sharma, "Trends in End-of-Life ICU Care among Older Adults with Advanced Lung Cancer," *Chest* 133, no. 1 (2008): 72–78; A. Kelley, "Determinants of Medical Expenditures in the Last Six Months of Life," *Annals of Internal Medicine* 154 (2011): 235–42; S. Kaufman, "Making Longevity in an Aging Society: Linking Ethical Sensibility and Medicare Spending," *Medical Anthropology* 28, no. 4 (2009): 317–25.

17. B. Jennings, "Health Care Costs in End-of-Life and Palliative Care: The Quest for Ethical Reform," *Journal of Social Work* 7 (2011): 300–317; Duggan, *Breaking the Iron Triangle*, 80.

18. Brownlee, *Overtreated*, 115; R. S. Pritchard, "Influence of Patient Preferences and Local Health System Characteristics on the Place of Death," *Journal of the American Geriatrics Society* 46 (1995): 1242–50; See notes XX–XX in chapter 1.

19. Brownlee, *Overtreated*, 49, 59, 113.

20. "Clinical Effectiveness: Community-Acquired Pneumonia," Texas Medical Association, http://www.texmed.org/community_acquired_pneumonia.aspx.

21. K. D. Frick, "Substitutive Hospital at Home for Older Persons: Effect on Costs," *American Journal of Managed Care* 15, no. 1 (2009): 49–56.

22. Byock, *Best Care Possible*, 233.

23. "Total Pay for Top Executives at Maryland Hospitals and Health Systems," *Baltimore Sun*, 2012, http://data.baltimoresun.com/from-cms/total-compensation-for-maryland-hospital-ceos-and-presidents-2012/.

24. American Hospital Association, "The Economic Contribution of Hospitals," http://www.aha.org/research/reports/13econimpact.shtml.

25. "Traditional Hospital Care vs. ACE Units for Geriatric Patients," Office of Geriatrics and Gerontology, Ohio State University Wexner Medical Center, 2013, https://ogg.osu.edu/newsletters/22/articles/90.

26. M. T. Fox, "Effectiveness of Acute Geriatric Unit Care Using Acute Care for Elders Components: A Systematic Review and Met Analysis," *Journal of the American Geriatrics Society* 60, no. 12 (2012): 2237–45; S. Counsell, "Effects of a Multicomponent Intervention on Functional Outcomes and Process of Care in Hospitalized Older Patients: A Randomized Controlled Trial of Acute Care for Elders (ACE) in a Community Hospital," *Journal of the American Geriatrics Society* 48, no. 12 (2000): 1572–81.

27. K. Flood, "Effect of an Acute Care for Elders Unit on Costs and Thirty-Day Readmissions," *JAMA Internal Medicine* 173, no. 11 (June 2013): 981–87.

28. Senior Services, Holy Cross Health, http://www.holycrosshealth.org/seniors-emergency-centers.

29. U. Hwang, "The Geriatric Emergency Department," *Journal of the American Geriatrics Society* 55, no. 11 (2007): 1873–76.

30. Byock, *Best Care Possible*, 112, 230.

5. Long-Term Care

1. Nortin Hadler, *Rethinking Aging* (Chapel Hill: University of North Carolina Press, 2011), 171.

2. K. Walshe, "Regulating US Nursing Homes: Are We Learning from Experience?" *Health Affairs* 20, no. 6 (2001): 128–44; J. Troyer, "The Impact of Litigation on Nursing Home Quality," *Journal of Health Politics, Policy, and Law* 29, no. 1 (2004): 11–42.

3. M. Gillick, "Rethinking the Role of Tube Feeds in Patients with Advanced Dementia," *New England Journal of Medicine* 342 (2000): 206–10; M. Kau, "Long-Term Follow-Up of Consequences of PEG Tubes in Nursing Home Patients," *Digestive Disease and Science* 39, no. 4 (1994): 738–43; S. Mitchell, "The Risk Factors and Impact on Survival of Feeding Tube Placement in Nursing Home Residents with Severe Cognitive Impairment," *Archives of Internal Medicine* 157, no. 3 (1997): 327–32.

4. L. Rubenstein, "Falls in the Nursing Home," *Annals of Internal Medicine* 121, no. 6 (1994): 442–51; L. Lipsitz, "Cause and Correlates of Recurrent Falls in Ambulatory Frail Elderly," *Journal of Gerontology* 46, no. 4 (1991): 114–22; L. Rubenstein, "Falls and Fall Prevention in the Nursing Home," *Clinics in Geriatric Medicine* 12, no. 4 (1996): 881–902.

5. John Abramson, *Overdosed America: The Broken Promise of American Medicine* (New York: Harpers, 2008), 218.

6. J. Cohen-Mansfield, "Turnover among Nursing Home Staff: A Review," *Nurse Manager* 28, no. 5 (1997): 59–64; N. Castle, "Staff Turnover and Quality of Care in Nursing Homes," *Medical Care* 43, no. 6 (2005): 616–26.

7. C. Harrington, "Nursing Home Staffing and Its Relationship to Deficiencies," *Journal of Gerontology* 55, no. 5 (2000): 278–87.

8. R. L. Kruse, "Does Hospitalization Impact Survival after Lower Respiratory Infection in Nursing Home Residents?" *Medical Care* 42 (2004): 860–70; M. Loeb, "Effect of a Clinical Pathway to Reduce Hospitalization in Nursing Home Residents with Pneumonia," *Journal of the American Medical Association* 295, no. 21 (June 2006): 2503–10; J. L. Givens, "Survival and Comfort after Treatment of Pneumonia in Advanced Dementia," *Archives of Internal Medicine* 171, no. 3 (2011): 217.

9. P. Gozalo, "End-of-Life Transitions among Nursing Home Residents with Cognitive Issues," *New England Journal of Medicine* 365 (2011): 1212–21.

10. A. J. Forster, "The Incidence and Severity of Adverse Effects Affecting Patients after Discharge from the Hospital," *Annals of Internal Medicine* 138 (2003): 161–67; K. Boockvar, "Adverse Effects Due to Discontinuations in Drug Use and Dose Change in Patients Transferred between Acute and Long-Term Facilities," *Archives of Internal Medicine* 164, no. 5 (2004): 545–50.

11. D. Steunser, "The Rise of Nursing Home Litigation: Findings from a National Survey of Attorneys," *Health Affairs* 22, no. 2 (2003): 219–29.

12. M. Kapp, "Nursing Home Culture Change: Legal Apprehensions and Opportunities," *Gerontologist* 53, no. 5 (2013): 718–26.

13. Gozalo, "End-of-Life Transitions."

14. T. Fried, "Fragility and Hospitalization of Long Term Stay Nursing Home Residents," *Journal of the American Geriatric Society* 45, no. 3 (1997): 265–69.

15. O. Intrator, "Facility Characteristics Associated with Hospitalization of Nursing Home Residents: Results of a National Study," *Medical Care* 37, no. 3 (1999): 228–37.

16. Ibid.

17. Ira Byock, *The Best Care Possible* (New York: Avery, 2012), 45.

18. A. Grunier, "Hospitalization of Nursing Home Residents with Cognitive Impairments: The Influence of Organizational Features and State Policies," *Gerontologist* 47 (2007): 447–56.

19. Byock, *Best Care Possible*, 103, 112.

20. Medpac, "Report to the Congress: Medicare Payment Policy," March 2015, 289, http://www.medpac.gov/documents/reports/chapter-12-hospice-services-(march-2015-report).pdf?sfvrsn=0.

21. Jordan Rau, "Concerns about Costs Rise with Hospices' Use," *New York Times,* June 28, 2011, D1.

22. P. Whoriskey, "In Hospice, but Not Dying," *Washington Post*, December 27, 2013, 1.

23. "Nursing Home or Hospital: The Medical Director's Response to Increasing Medical Acuity," AMDA Long-Term Care Conference, March 21–24, 2013.

6. Quality and Value

1. S. Burwell, "Setting Value-Based Payment Goals: HHS Efforts to Improve U.S. Health Care," *New England Journal of Medicine* 372 (2015): 897–99.

2. J. Tozzi, "The Problem with Obama's Plan to Pay Doctors Based on Performance," *Bloomberg Politics*, May 8, 2015.

3. V. Prasad, "President Bush's Unnecessary Surgery," *Washington Post*, August 9, 2013, A23.

4. M. Hendrickson, "Did You Really Pay for Your Medicare Benefits?" *Forbes*, March 7, 2013, http://www.forbes.com/sites/markhendrickson/2013/03/07/did-you-really-pay-for-your-medicare-benefits/.

5. Shannon Brownlee, *Overtreated: Why Too Much Medicine Is Making Us Sicker and Poorer* (New York: Bloomsbury Press, 2007), 269–87.

6. Z. Meisel and J. Pines, "Post-HMO Health Care: Are ACOs the Answer?" *Time*, May 31, 2011, http://content.time.com/time/health/article/0,8599,2074816,00.html.

7. John Abramson, *Overdosed America: The Broken Promise of American Medicine* (New York: Harpers, 2008), 81; D. C. Angus, "The Effect of Managed Care on ICU Length of Stay: Implications for Medicare," *Journal of the American Medical Association* 276, no. 13 (October 1996): 1075–82.

8. A. Gawande, "Overkill." *The New Yorker,* May 11, 2015.

9. Stephen Schimpff, *Fixing the Primary Care Crisis: Reclaiming the Patient-Doctor Relationship and Returning Healthcare Decisions to You and Your Doctor* (Createspace, 2015).

10. S. Boodman, "The 1% Solution," *Washington Post*, October 18, 2013, E1.

11. J. Hancock, "Health-Law Test to Cut Readmissions Lacks Early Results," *Kaiser Health News*, January 14, 2015.

12. The CMS Innovation Center, http://www.innovation.cms.gov.

13. "Affordable Care Act," US Department of Health and Human Services, http://www.hhs.gov/opa/affordable-care-act/index.html.

14. L. Zamosky, "Will a New Anti-Fraud Campaign Lead to More Audits?" *Medical Economics*, October 25, 2013, http://www.physicianspractice.com/blog/six-main-reasons-physicians-are-dropping-medicare-patients.

15. "Do Electronic Medical Records Save Money?" *New York Times*, editorial, March 6, 2012; S. Kliff, "Why Electronic Health Records Failed," *Washington Post*, January 11, 2013.

16. J. Rau, "Medicare Is Stingy in First Year of Doctor Bonuses," *Kaiser Health News,* April 6, 2015.

17. B. Japsen, "Half of US Patients Can Access Obamacare's 'Accountable Care Organizations,'" February 18, 2013, *Forbes*, http://www.forbes.com/sites/brucejapsen/2013/02/18/half-of-u-s-patients-can-access-obamacares-accountable-care-organizations/.

18. Northern Maryland Collaborative Care, *Provider Handbook*, http://www.northernmdcc.com.

19. M. McClellan and S. Kocot, "Early Evidence on Medicare ACOs and Next Steps," *Health Affairs Blog*, January 22, 2015.

20. S. Heiser and C. Colla, "Unpacking the Medicare Shared Savings Proposed Rule," *Health Affairs Blog*, January 22, 2015.

21. AMDA Long Term Care Conference, 3/21–3/24, 2013: D. Adams, "ACOs: Payer Driven Innovations in LTC," and J. Nichols, "What a Medical Director Needs to Know about Bundled Payments and ACOs."

22. J. Rau, "Medicare Speeds Up Pay Plan," *Washington Post*, July 22, 2013, A15.

23. N. Doughler, "Can Accountable Care Organizations Improve Population Health?" *Journal of the American Medical Association* 309, no. 111 (March 2013): 119.

24. B. Landon, "Keeping Score under a Global Payment System," *New England Journal of Medicine* 366 (2012): 393–95.

25. D. Rittenhouse, "Primary Care and Accountable Care: Two Essential Elements of Delivery-System Reform," *New England Journal of Medicine* 361 (2009): 2301–3.

26. L. Burns, "Accountable Care Organizations May Have Difficulty Avoiding the Failures of Integrative Delivery Networks of the 1990s," *Health Affairs* 31, no. 11 (2012): 2407–16.

27. J. Hancock, "Mixed Results for Obamacare Test in Primary Care Innovation," *Kaiser Health News,* January 30, 2015.

28. S. London, "Pioneer ACO Model Cuts Medicare Costs, Receives Certification," Medscape Medical News, May 4, 2015.

29. "Diagnosis-Related Group," Wikipedia, https://en.wikipedia.org/wiki/Diagnosis-related_group.

30. J. Ezekiel, "Saving by the Bundle," *New York Times*, November 16, 2011.

31. W. Weeks, "The Unintended Consequences of Bundled Payments," *Annals of Internal Medicine* 158, no. 1 (2013): 62–64.

32. M. Naylor, "Unintended Consequences of Steps to Cut Readmissions and Reform Payment May Threaten Care of Vulnerable Older Adults," *Health Affairs* 31, no. 7 (2012): 1023–36.

33. AAMC, "Independent Payment Advisory Board," http://www.aamc.org/advocacy/medicare/153896/independent-payment-advisory-board_ipab.html.

34. H. Dean, "The ACAs Rate Setting Won't Work," *Wall Street Journal*, July 28, 2013.

35. Peter R. Orszag, "The Critics Are Wrong about IPAB," *The Health Care Blog*, July 31, 2013, http://thehealthcareblog.com/blog/2013/07/31/the-critics-are-wrong-about-ipab/.

36. R. Lowes, "Bill to Repeal IPAB Gaining Momentum," Medscape Medical News, May 11, 2015.

37. C. Vestal, "Maryland May Be the Model for Curbing Hospital Costs," *USA Today*, January 31, 2014, http://www.usatoday.com/story/news/nation/2014/01/31/stateline-maryland-hospital-costs/5079073.

38. S. Gottleib, "The Doctor Won't See You Now. He's Closed," *Wall Street Journal,* January 14, 2013; L. Osby, "Hospitals Buying More Doctors' Practices," *USA Today*, September 14, 2013.

39. G. C. Alexander and E. Keyes, "The Best Medicine: A Good Relationship with Your Doc," *Baltimore Sun,* May 7, 2015.

40. O. Wengwarth and G. Gigerenzer, "Less Is More: Overdiagnosis and Overtreatment: Evaluation of What Physicians Tell Their Patients about Screening Harms," *JAMA Internal Medicine* 173, no. 22 (2013): 2086–87.

41. J. Hersch and A. Barratt, "Use of a Decision Aid Including Information on Overdetection to Support Informed Choice about Breast Cancer Screening: A Randomized Controlled Trial," *Lancet,* February 17, 2015.

42. E. Rifkin and A. Lazris, *Interpreting Health Benefits and Risks: A Practical Guide to Facilitate Doctor-Patient Communication.* Switzerland: Springer International Publishing, 2015.

43. "A Hopeful Vote on Medicare," *Washington Post*, April 17, 2015, A18.

44. M. Crane, "Doctors Applaud SGR Bill's Malpractice Protection," Medscape Internal Medicine, April 16, 2015.

45. P. Gozalo and M. Plozke, "Changes in Medicare Costs with the Growth of Hospice Care in Nursing Homes," *New England Journal of Medicine* 372 (2015): 1823–31.

46. D. Meier, "Increased Access to Palliative Care and Hospice Services: Opportunities to Improve Value in Health Care," *Milbank Quarterly* 89, no. 3 (September 2011): 343–80.

47. A. Bazemore and S. Petterson, "More Comprehensive Care among Family Physicians Is Associated with Lower Costs and Fewer Hospitalizations," *Annals of Family Medicine* 13, no. 3 (May/June 2015): 206–13.

48. Daniela Drake, "The Health-Care System Is So Broken, It's Time for Doctors to Strike," *The Daily Beast*, April 29, 2014, http://www.thedailybeast.com/articles/2014/04/29/the-health-care-system-is-so-broken-it-s-time-for-doctors-to-strike.html; Daniela Drake, "How Being a Doctor Became the Most Miserable Profession," *The Daily Beast*, April 14, 2014, http://www.thedailybeast.com/articles/2014/04/14/how-being-a-doctor-became-the-most-miserable-profession.html.

49. D. Muller, "Reforming Premedical Education: Out with the Old, In with the New," *New England Journal of Medicine* 368 (2013): 1567–69.

50. C. Rampell, "How Medicare Subsidizes Doctor Training," *New York Times,* December 17, 2013.

51. A. Otani, "Med School Deans Worry Graduates Won't Get Residencies," *Bloomberg Business,* May 11, 2015.

52. E. Emanuel, "Shortening Medical Training by 30%," *Journal of the American Medical Association* 307, no. 11 (March 2012): 1043–44.

53. S. Boodman, "Fast Track through Medical School," *Washington Post*, January 14, 2014, E1.

Afterword

1. J. Verghese, "Leisure Activities and the Risk of Dementia in the Elderly," *New England Journal of Medicine* 348 (2003): 2508–16; E. W. Gregg, "Relationship of Changes in Physical Activity and Mortality among Older Women," *Journal of the American Medical Association* 289, no. 18 (May 2003): 2379–86; N. T. Lautenschlage, "Effect of Physical Activity on Cognitive Function in Older Adults at Risk of Alzheimer's Disease," *Journal of the American Medical Association* 300, no. 9 (October 2008): 1027–37; E. Larson, "Exercise Is Associated with Reduced Risk for Incident Dementia among Persons 65 Years of Age and Older," *Annals of Internal Medicine* 144, no. 2 (2006): 73–81. Many more similar studies are published frequently.

Index

Page numbers in *italics* indicate figures.

A1C sugar level, 31–32, 94–95
abdominal aortic aneurysm (AAA), 63–64
absolute risk and benefit, 23–27, 35, 61–63, 91, 195
academic physicians, 11, 41, 42, 47, 48, 82, 100
accountable care organizations (ACOs), 19, 47–48, 103–4, 174, 179–83, 186–87, 202
ACE (acute care for elders) units, 125
acid reflux, 36, 43
acute care, xi, 95, 123–25, 184, 200
advanced directives, x, 150, 158
advertising, 38, 40–44
Affordable Care Act (ACA), 6, 43, 88, 124, 169, 201–3; clinical guidelines, 47–48; Medicare reform and, 172–75
aggressive care: belief in, 5, 14–15; death caused by, x, 16, 20–21, 49, 72–73, 76, 77; defensive medicine, 105–6; families pressured into, 145–47; hospitalization and, 113–17; long-term care and, 129–30, 157–58; Medicare payment for, 57, 72–73, 76–78, 83; patients as victims of, 2–3
aging: as disease, 22, 45, 50, 103; misunderstanding of, 15–16; natural declines, 53, 54; stress and inactivity as enemies of, 212; stress-free, 12–13
agitated patients, xii, 2, 137, 140, 142–43
alendronate (Fosamax), 35–36
alternative payment models, 165
Alzheimer's, 7–8, 39, 81, 82
AMDA conference, 161–62, 181
American Hospital Association, 125
American Medical Association (AMA), ix–x, 7, 102–3
American Medical Association Board, 97